The Hospice
Movement

THE HOSPICE MOVEMENT

A Better Way of Caring for the Dying

Sandol Stoddard

STEIN AND DAY/PUBLISHERS

First published in 1978
Copyright © 1978 by Sandol Stoddard
All rights reserved
Designed by Leonard Telesca
Printed in the United States of America
Stein and Day/*Publishers*/Scarborough House, Briarcliff Manor, N.Y. 10510

SECOND PRINTING, 1978

"Pain has an Element of Blank" by Emily Dickinson is reprinted by permission of the publishers and the Trustees of Amherst College from THE POEMS OF EMILY DICKINSON, edited by Thomas H. Johnson, Cambridge, Mass.: The Belknap Press of Harvard University Press, Copyright © 1951, 1955 by the President and Fellows of Harvard College.

Library of Congress Cataloging in Publication Data

Stoddard, Sandol
    The Hospice movement.

    1. Terminal care. 2. Terminal care facilities. 3. History of Hospitals
I. Title.
R726.8.W37   616   77-2951
ISBN 0-8128-2178-5

To
CFS — CHS
and all
who
have given me life

Acknowledgments

My debts are many, to friends and colleagues, and to professionals in various fields who have read this book in manuscript, lending me their guidance and their criticism as well as their encouragement. It is usual to say, but I would like to say it with special emphasis in this case, that any errors of fact or judgment which may nevertheless appear here are definitely my own. As each person listed below knows very well, I am not in the habit of taking at all times even the very best of advice.

Dr. Cicely Saunders has read and reread revisions of the work chapter by chapter as it emerged, offering corrections, additions, and suggestions at many points, and lending to the entire project the nurturing power of her remarkable mind and spirit. For this I am deeply grateful, and equally so for the fact that she gave me the inestimable joy and privilege of working with patients at St. Christopher's Hospice, London.

Dr. Gert Brieger, Chairman of the Department of the History of Health Sciences at the University of California, San Francisco, has greatly honored me by taking time to read the entire manuscript, has suggested a number of improvements, and has delighted me with the wit and perceptiveness of his comments at every point.

Dr. Matthew Evans, Chairman of the Department of Humanities at San Francisco State University, showed me many years ago the source of the hospice movement. His reading of this manuscript has served throughout the process of revision, not only to renew my sense of purpose (and of gratitude), but to guide me on the narrow path between bogs of sense and quicksands of sentiment. For whatever measure of safe deliverance I may have achieved, he is to be heartily thanked.

Dr. Donald T. Kishi, Pharm. D., Associate Clinical Professor of Pharmacy at the University of California, San Francisco, has been most kind in preparing the "translations" of British medicines into their American equivalents. Mr. Charles H. G. O'Gara has my gratitude for his assistance in connection with the grant from the S. K. Wellman Foundation, Inc., of Cleveland, Ohio, which was so important an aid to the research done abroad.

I am thankful to the many hospice directors and staff members who have given their time and energy in support of my research, especially Dr. William M. Lamers, Jr., who has provided, month after month, every sort of nourishment a writer needs. Dr. Sylvia Lack and Dr. R. G. Twycross have also been particularly generous in their assistance, and special thanks are due as well to Matron Helen Willans of St. Christopher's Hospice, whose peerless example as a hospice worker has been an inspiration to me throughout the writing of this book. To the patients who shared their lives with me, and to their families, I owe the debts of love which can never be repaid.

Help and advice, criticism, information, and encouragement have been received along the way from so many individuals that it is impossible to list them all here; but some mention must be made of my gratitude to Marcia Higgins, Zoila Schoenbrun, Dr. Richard Schoenbrun, Phyllis Atwood Watts, Joan Erikson, Caroline Leibert, Hilary Belloc, Margaret Frings Keyes, Paul Brooks, Dr. Maynard Mack, Georgina Battiscombe, Rev. Iain Wilson, Joan Corbett, Joanne Hively, Lee Adams, Rev. Frank Potter, Felix Knauth, James and Tally Harmon, Patricia Douglas, Joy Sweet, and August Brooks. My friend Janice Roberts, who died of cancer on April 29, 1977, gave me her strength in daily telephone calls of encouragement until that very date, and then scolded me for coming to her bedside at a time when, in her opinion, I should have been at home finishing Chapter 10.

To Father John Thornton, priest, friend and fellow-writer, I owe the debt that he alone knows, or could adequately express.

For her trust and patience, as well as her sensitive guidance, I am deeply grateful to my editor, Michaela Hamilton.

I thank the members of my family for their constant love and encouragement: Anthony and Judith, Peter and Melinda, Gerald and Deborah, and especially my son Jason, who has had to live with me while I was working on the book. Above all, I thank my husband and fellow-pilgrim, William Ames Atchley, physician and Clinical Professor of Medicine, who has carried me through thorn and briar while helping to light my way; who has "cherysshed and refreshed" beyond measure this entire work, and its author entirely.

Phoenix, Arizona
July 20, 1977

Contents

A Personal Foreword

Twenty-five years ago I lay in the large maternity hall of a respectable old Boston hospital, laboring to give birth to my first child. The name of the institution was world-famous, and the care given its lying-in patients was considered exemplary.

All around me in this vast, echoing room were beds with strips of canvas at the sides designed to keep unconscious or delirious patients from falling out. In these criblike structures, rows of women lay still as death, or tossed and moaned, or cried out for help or for water, or shrieked like victims on the rack. In accordance with the system of the day, the majority were heavily sedated. Few had any real understanding of what was happening. Women did not "get pregnant" in those days; at least, in middle-class New England they did not. They were found to be "having a baby" and the actual process of getting it born was seldom, if ever, discussed.

The babies arrived slowly. Most were taken by instruments at the obstetrician's convenience, for he was a busy man. My own obstetrician was one of the finest. He was so busy that it cost $1,000 every time he crossed the street from his office, washed his hands, and pulled a baby out of its mother's body with a pair of forceps. A thousand dollars was a great deal of money in those days. But of course, in matters of life and death, nothing but the best would do. Our babies arrived smelling of ether, listless and bruised, their heads dented like windfallen fruit.

xiv   *Sandol Stoddard*

In the bed beside mine all this long day and into the night, a young woman wept for her mother. I could see her long, dark hair lying in a tangle on the pillow. I remember thinking that she must be a visitor from some exotic land—France or Spain, or Italy perhaps—because when she was not crying out for her·mother, she was sobbing, *"Jesus, Jesus."*

Eventually her cries became piercingly loud and incessant. The two nurses on duty shrugged at one another in distaste, inspected her briefly, and decided to wheel her bed into a soundproof anteroom.

"Why don't you do something to help her?" I asked. "She is frightened out of her wits, and she is in terrible pain."

The nurses stared at me in consternation. "What are you doing awake?" asked one. "She isn't feeling anything. She is very heavily sedated."

"But listen to her," I insisted. "If she is not suffering, why is she screaming and begging for help?" The two nurses looked at one another, and looked away. "She'll forget about it soon enough," I was told. Then I was given an injection; and after that, I don't remember anything that happened to me for fourteen hours.

Many years later I lay resting comfortably in a very different sort of hospital, an institution also highly respected, and noted for its enlightened maternity care. My airy room overlooked the grassy, moonlit spaces of northern California on a summer night. Wide awake that afternoon, I had given birth to another child.

In a round mirror I had watched the crowning of the small, dark head. I had seen the eyes of the doctors and the nurses in attendance—caring, helping, encouraging, congratulating me. Family and friends had come to embrace me. Now I had flowers, music, wine, perfume and the silence of the night around me as I lay in a state of happiness so profound that sleep was irrelevant.

The day had been hard. The birth had been complicated and dangerous. I had been badly frightened, and had felt at times a great deal of pain. Yet, with the help of those around me, I had been able to obey the enormous demand of that primal event.

And in doing so, I had experienced a new dimension of reality. Claiming a birthright of my own, I had journeyed that day to a place beyond pain or death. Heaven, some would say, had opened itself to me.

A mystical moment, others might call it, or "a peak experience"—that glimpse of a joy beyond joy or grief, of a great reconciliation shining at the heart of things. At any rate, I knew that as long as I lived I could never be afraid of dying again. Dying and giving birth, being born and dying: in some inexplicable way, I had come to know that they are the same.

As I lay there, perfectly comforted and at peace, I began to hear on the other side of the wall beside me the voice of a woman weeping. *"God! Oh, God,"* she cried, and then I heard her calling for her mother. Poor love, I thought. Soon it will be better, you'll see. I could hear her struggling for breath, grappling, laboring. Another child coming into the world, I thought—the wonder of it, the mystery! She began to scream, "I can't do it! I can't!" Oh, my dear, I thought, yes you can—but why on earth doesn't anyone come to help you? I rang my own bell.

Footsteps. Doors opening and closing. Voices. A telephone ringing. Beyond the wall, the sobbing and the moaning, on and on.

I tried to get out of my bed, and found that I was too weak. Through the wall, then, I tried somehow to lend her what energy I had. *Don't be afraid,* I thought. *Just breathe, in and out, and then, let go.* "Oh God!" she began to scream again. *Let go,* I thought, *let go.*

Footsteps again, and the night nurse was standing over me. "What are you doing awake?" she scolded. Beyond the wall, the screams continued. "Don't worry about her," the nurse said hastily. "She isn't suffering. She is very heavily sedated."

"But why . . . ?"

"Don't worry about it," said the nurse.

"But no one goes to her," I said. "Why doesn't anyone go in there and try to help her?"

"It wouldn't make any difference," replied the nurse, giving me an injection. "She doesn't know what she is doing. If it bothers you, dear, just turn up your radio."

Early in the morning I awakened and crept out of my bed. I made my way to the room next door. It was empty, and the bed was stripped. It took me two more days to find out what had been happening in that room. Everyone I asked about it was either disinterested or embarrassed.

I made a nuisance of myself until at last it was explained. There had been an administrative error. The person in question, a female aged thirty-seven, Caucasian, single, had not been giving birth; she had been dying. She had no business to be in the maternity department. She was cancer, terminal.

The patient had been in the hospital many times before, they told me. There was nothing more anyone could do for her. They had already cut out her breasts, her ovaries, her uterus. She had lost her eyesight, her fingernails, her hair. She was incontinent, and even when fully conscious, she was not altogether in her right mind. She belonged in medical-surgical, obviously.

For nine days before the birth of my child, they had been trying to get her moved. At first her papers had been misfiled, and then there had been a problem about insurance. After that, there had simply been no other place for her to go. Under ordinary circumstances they would have put her, when she was being so noisy, into the little isolation cubicle behind the nursery. As it happened, even that room at the time had been filled.

They were terribly sorry. The whole thing had been very unfortunate. They apologized to me for the inconvenience I had suffered, having to lie awake next door to her and, due to the poor quality of the soundproofing of that wing, having to listen to her die.

The faces of the individuals who said these things to me were somewhat puzzled and distracted, but they were not cruel or even unkind. In fact, I have rarely found medical people—or people of any sort—to be deliberately stupid or consciously mean and enjoying it. Still, it is hard to reply to well-intentioned people who are, in matters of life and death, so very far off the mark. It has taken me some time to find a useful way of responding to the experiences I have here described.

In part, this book is my response. And although it contains a good deal of history and many facts about death and loss, it is nevertheless a celebration of life.

"After a long illness ... at a local hospital ..." is what the newspapers say. Someone anonymous, it seems, is always dying while the rest of us turn up the radio or look the other way. And yet, having accepted the realities of birth as a natural process to be celebrated and respected, we are now bound, I think, to have a clearer look at the process of death.

In medieval times, dying persons were seen as prophetic souls, voyagers and pilgrims valuable to the community in a number of ways, not least in the opportunity they provided those around them for service and spiritual growth. It is a modern and ignorant prejudice to consider death a failure. It is a modern superstition to avoid knowledge of it, to treat it as if it were something unnatural, shameful, or wrong.

It is time for us to root out the fears and misconceptions that lie behind this distorted view. We must begin to honor the labor of those pilgrims who journey on before us; and in being present for them during the part of their living which is called dying, we must learn better to honor life itself.

This is what the hospice movement is all about. If my dying neighbor, Caucasian female aged thirty-seven, had been cared for in a hospice instead of a general hospital, she would not have been forsaken and she would not have been in agony at the hour of her death. She would in all probability have been spared some of the surgical degradations she was made to suffer in the name of "cure"—and she would have had a name. She would have been surrounded by people who knew and loved her. Her pain would have been honored and skillfully relieved. She would have mattered as a person, not as the anonymous receptacle of a disease. With hospice care, the woman whose name I will never know would have had safe lodging, and love, and peace at the last.

No one in a civilized society should have to die as she did. The emergence of the modern hospice in our world today brings with it the hope and, potentially, the promise of a far better way than this for all of us.

The Hospice
Movement

The Caring Host

CHAPTER 1

Hospice (ho'spis) [a.F. *hospice*, ad. L. *hospitium* hospitality, entertainment, a lodging, inn, f. *hospit-em:* see HOST sb^2] 1. A house of rest and entertainment for pilgrims, travellers or strangers . . . for the destitute or the sick.

Oxford English Dictionary

. . . For the ayde and comforte of the poore sykke, blynde, aged and impotent persones . . . whereyn they may be lodged, cherysshed and refreshed.

From a petition by the
citizens of London to
Henry VIII (1538)

It is 3 A.M. and the television set of the ordinary householder is turned off. Downtown, however, in the newest wing of the university hospital, a skilled RN scans another set of screens. In the sophisticated purlieus of the intensive care unit, the drama is complex, intense, continuous. Here the humblest, least conspicuous of human signals is translated instantly into a series of extraordinary elegant mechanical events. The ICU is a supercomputer, a biochemical celebration, a sound-and-light show. It is also something like a launching pad. Disconnected from every familiar form of human contact and every ordinary support system, the patients lie one by one, espaliered, wired, and tuned like astronauts. In the silence of the night it might be asked—where are they going? But in this place there is no silence, and there is no night.

In places of transit—bus stations, train stations, space stations, airports, hotels, hospitals—lights blaze twenty-four hours a day. Surfaces are hard here, cold and glittering; there is a smell of disinfectant in the air. People in such environs experience loneliness, anxiety, disorientation, a loss of the sense of personal identity. They become part of a mechanical situation, an observed and measured event.

Bus stations, space stations, hotels, hospitals. Question: does the word *hotel* belong in this group? If you have felt the urge to cross it out, then you may be one of the fortunate—one of the lucky few—who remember what the deliciously intimate hotels of the world used to be like before they, too, began wrapping the facilities in paper and the drinking glasses (for your protection) in plastic. Or perhaps you remember with delight those little places in Paris which until recently, that is to say, until a century or so ago, have been private homes. The curtains hang in shreds, there are mouse-tracks under the armoire, and the bed squeaks—but the hospitable concierge slips you a wink and an extra croissant with your morning chocolate; and every room is filled with roses.

The Latin word *hospes* meant both host and guest. This in itself is interesting, since it puts the spotlight on a process, an interaction between human beings, which was once perceived as simple and mutual. In terms of our present medical models, both as promoted in the media and as experienced in professional practice, it is even more fascinating to consider the development of the word *hospes* into *hospitium,* into *hostel, hôtel-Dieu* and *hospice;* also, of course, into *host* and *hostess,* into *hotel, motel,* and *hospital.* It is a sort of litany we have here, recording subtle shifts in value judgments, and in the differing relationships people have chosen, over the centuries, to have with one another. It is a litany perhaps worthy of some contemplation.

Certainly it is a measure, for example, of the split between mind and heart in the modern consciousness that we have needed a dictionary to help us recover the ancient connection between the objective thing, *hospital,* and the embracing act, *hospitality.*

It is a strange embrace, the one we now find welcoming us into the place called *hospital.* It is one which neutralizes instantly whatever life force it is that makes each one of us into a unique individual. *Hospital* welcomes my body as so many pounds of meat, filled with potentially interesting mechanical parts and neurochemical combinations. *Hospital* strips me of all personal privacy, of all sensual pleasure, of every joy the soul finds delight in; and at the same time, seizes me in the intimacy of a total embrace. *Hospital* makes war, not love.

Let us leave sentimentality out of it, by all means. Sentimentality is more life-destroying than honest hate. The sentimental host does no good to me; he only calls attention to his own needs without looking after mine. My need, if I am very ill, and especially if I am on the point of dying, is not for sappy get-well cards and background music. If there is a chance of mending me, so much the better. For example, that flesh wound I picked up during a difference of opinion with a would-be mugger: I very much appreciate having my host, the intern, sew it up for me. He need not be a television star. If he prevents me from bleeding to death as the result of a senseless assault, he looks beautiful to me. I am delighted to have my heart started up again by technicians of any sort, using whatever means they may have at their disposal, if my heart has quit simply because I overburdened it with carrying packages on a hot day. I will gladly be their guest, I am grateful for their assistance, and none of us needs to get teary-eyed over the drama of it all.

And yet, hardboiled, practical, and ruthlessly realistic as we in the modern medical situation may imagine ourselves to be, is it not incredibly *sentimental* for us to imagine that we are engaged all this time in conquering an enemy called Death? Our young medical soldiers in the media are so brave, so attractive, one wants them always to win. There is a mystique about this war against death that makes us turn our heads away from those who are hopelessly, incurably ill; and also from those who are quite consciously ready to die. These are the ones who disturb our picture of the way things ought to be. From *hospes* to *hospital,* the psychology has changed from one of love to one of war, and in the psychology of war, force is imperative. Therefore we arrive at the strange, new embrace that pins the inert body of a man or woman, terminally ill, to a machine which forces that person's body to breathe without even knowing its name.

It is our attitude toward death, I believe, that has so badly skewed and spoiled our contemporary sense of how persons who are well ought to relate to persons who are sick. In America, for reasons having to do with the development of our own culture, the problem is particularly acute.

"Death is un-American," Arnold Toynbee once remarked. It denies our power to conquer the globe with know-how and muscle, with science and machinery, with the youthful vigor and hope that conquered the frontier. Mocking what we have unconsciously believed was our inalienable right to live happily ever after, the Grim Reaper still awaits us at the end of every path we launch into the wilderness, or into space. The death of a patient is perceived as a humiliation and an outrage by the average physician in our culture; to the nursing staff in an acute-care hospital, it feels like a personal defeat. To the patient's family it may very well represent the occasion for a malpractice suit. For indeed, why should such an untoward thing as death be allowed to happen in our society? The very look of a modern hospital identifies it as a fortress, an armory, a place of battle. The doctors dressed for combat with their engines and their weapons of cold steel—are they not the Knights Errant of our modern Crusades? If death succeeds in storming such walls as these, who has been at fault? Who has slept on watch? Or, has there been a traitor within?

Medical Nemesis, a recent book by Marxist theoretician Ivan Illich, has sought to capitalize, if I am not mistaken, upon the very real pain of this dilemma. It is not comfortable to live with a myth that isn't working, and Illich claims to have caught us all in the act of worshipping our doctors as if they were infallible shamans and sorcerers. The fact is, the secret has been out for some time that they are far from omnipotent. Our discomfort at the thought has long ago turned to rage, and we call regularly now upon attorneys to punish our former idols in the courts, much as Polynesian natives of the eighteenth century beat their tikis to a pulp when these objects of worship failed to perform as expected. The attempt of Illich and a number of other recent writers to ride this wave of anger is not really very enlightening to the public. What is needed instead, is a better grasp of the problem as a whole, and a set of new alternatives for coping with it. Physicians themselves, as we will see in the present study, are in the forefront of a movement to accomplish this very purpose.

The unadorned truth is that of 4.1 billion human beings alive on this planet at the moment, some 70 million of us will die this year despite the best and the worst that the medical profession can do. Yet all of this takes place, as Lewis Thomas reminds us, "... in relative secrecy. We can only really know of the deaths in our own households, or among our friends. These, detached in our minds from all the rest, we take to be unnatural events, anomalies, outrages. We speak of our own dead in low voices; struck down, we say, as though visible death can only occur for cause, by disease or violence, avoidably." Death will happen to us all, and will happen because in the natural order of things, it is supposed to happen. That is the unsentimental fact of the matter, the fact undistorted by myth or imagination. It is also a *hospitable* fact, come to think of it. Moving over, leaving space for someone else to have a chance: why shouldn't I be required to do this, as well as anyone else?

Unfortunately, just as we have lost the conscious connection between the word *hospital* and the word *hospitality*, we have also managed to lose a sense of the proper, necessary, and positive continuity between life and death. For too long a time we have maintained a really unfortunate illusion that one can exist without the other.

A new wave of awareness is beginning at last to change all of this in some positive ways. Pioneers such as Dr. Cicely Saunders in England and Dr. Elisabeth Kübler-Ross in the United States have brought the subject of dying into the open, and have helped us to learn more about the reality of it. Hundreds of books and articles have suddenly appeared in the past ten years, describing and analyzing the processes of death, dying, mourning, and bereavement. Courses, particularly in the United States, are being given in schools and colleges to help young people reach a better understanding of a subject that was, until very recently, taboo, Films have begun to appear (notably, Michael Roemer's magnificent documentary, *Dying*) that treat the subject sanely, with decent concern and respect, and with none of the mawkishness that has served so often in the past as a mask for fear. Improved communication with the terminally ill and enlightened care of their needs has become a topic of great and ever-increasing public interest.

We have begun to realize, I believe, that the enemy all along was not death, but our own unwillingness to incorporate its reality into our consciousness. There are a number of reasons why we have been able to do such a good job of deceiving ourselves over the past hundred or so years on this particular subject. In our present culture, more and more people are living a great deal longer than they used to. The dying are now more or less automatically removed from their traditional position as protagonists in a communal drama: the deathbed scene. They are whisked away to the medical fortress where machines instead of human beings will be their companions at the last. Even nursing homes for the aged and incurably ill tend to maintain the myth that no one actually dies there. They are called, as a rule, "convalescent homes" and dead inmates are rushed out the back door so as not to give the place a bad name. We have also the current worship of youth and youthful life-styles to contend with in a culture which has forgotten—temporarily, one hopes—how to nourish itself upon the experience of its elders. Last but not least, we have the chilly Puritan attitude that loss of individual power, vigor, and self-control is somehow disgusting: the same attitude that in the past has buried sex in the unconscious or else turned it into pornography, manageable because plastic and fake. In the Puritan system, orgasmic experience involving personal surrender of any sort must be denied, and therefore, after the late Middle Ages, says Philippe Aries ". . . like the sexual act, death was henceforth increasingly thought of as a transgression which tears man from his daily life, from rational society, from his monotonous work, in order to make him undergo a paroxysm plunging him into an irrational, violent and beautiful world."

Beautiful though the world of death may be—and we have some rather astonishing evidence on this score, which will be taken up in a later chapter—the experience of dying can be a very difficult one.

"Dying is hard work," says Dr. T. S. West of St. Christopher's Hospice in London. The woman who gives birth instantly and unexpectedly, in a taxicab perhaps, or in a public rest room; the man who, looking the other way, is smashed to bits by a truck; or, feeling a little overtired one morning, leans over to tie his shoes and is dead before he finishes—these, fortunately or unfortunately, are the exceptions among us. In most cases, dying, like birthing, is a process requiring assistance. It is an event that asks us to be present for one another with heart and mind, bringing not only practical help as necessary, but also attentive awareness and appreciation of the individual involved. At its finest, it elicits from us the frankly and fully offered human companionship that brings positive benefits, and a kind of joy, to any shared venture.

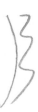

Oddly enough, most of this was known long ago, when the early medieval *hospice* was in operation throughout Europe, not only in England (where some 750 were counted at a time of minimum population) but in major towns and cities across the map (40 in Paris alone, 30 in Florence); at monastic hermitages in wilderness areas; and in particular, at the mountain passes and river crossings that presented the greatest hazards to travelers on their way to the Holy Land. It was natural enough in those days to see death as a venture, for life itself was perceived then as a journey, a pilgrimage. Man was not expected, in the days before the Renaissance, to be omnipotent. The ancient *hospice* differed from the modern *hospital* in many ways. It offered an open door of welcome not only to the sick and dying, but to the hungry wayfarer, the woman in labor, the needy poor, the orphan, or the leper with his bell. The common base or denominator of the offering was *hospitality* in its original sense of protection, refreshment, "cherysshing," and fellowship, rather than the demand of a patient for a cure.

Powerful herbs grew in the gardens of medieval, monastic hospices. Medieval medicine—and Greek, Egyptian, Indian, and

Babylonian medicine long before it—provided many a wise prescription for the healing of the body and the soul. Many are turning out today to be as effective as those we have discovered since. But it is the view of human value and of the human relationships involved that makes it most intriguing to study the development of the hospice from its earliest beginnings to the present day.

Endings and beginnings. Where does any idea or created thing ever really end, and where does it begin? "What are the Middle Ages?" asks medical historian David Riesman. "For all we know we may be living in them." The hospice idea did not begin with the work of Dr. Saunders in the 1960s, nor with the Irish Sisters of Charity in Dublin a hundred years before. It was not invented by the White Cross Knights of the eleventh century, nor by the Benedictines, nor did it have its beginnings with the rescue-dogs of Saint Bernard in the Alps. The concept antedates the magnificent hospice of Turmanin in Syria, A.D. 475 and the far more modest one founded in the port of Rome much earlier than that by a disciple of Saint Jerome named Fabiola, to care for pilgrims returning from Africa. Pilgrims returning from Africa— almost two thousand years ago! People traveled tremendous distances in those days, perhaps more boldly and freely than we are used to think.

It must have been a tremendous nuisance at times—people wandering in, as it would have been said in the old language, *per ager*, which means literally, *across the field*. Life was a struggle, in those days. If I live in my own village with wild animals in the woods all around me, I am likely to have my hands full keeping the fences mended, shearing my sheep, trying to raise a little barley and some oats, and keeping my chickens and my goat alive. I don't need foreigners and strangers *peregrinating* across the field, arriving tired and dirty just as my stew turns tender in the pot.

Or do I? It gets lonesome here, to tell you the truth, from time to time. If only I knew whether in some way or another this fellow might be useful to me, I might let him in. So, I try it. He likes it, and he stays. "Three days gast," says the ancient Anglo-Saxon law, and after that, *"agen hine."* The Anglo-Saxons were succinct. Plautus in 205 B.C. put it more elaborately, perhaps, but no less firmly: "After three days, a guest and a fish begin to stink."

And yet, with incredible persistence, the stranger kept coming over the field. I began to discover that he often brought me news that was helpful to me; sometimes he taught me some new skill, or enlarged my viewpoint one way or another about my own situation. If the person who came *per ager,* that is to say, the *peregrina,* fell ill while staying with me, I nursed him as best I could, without knowing quite why I did it; and if he died, I buried him.

Over the centuries then, there were times when I myself found reasons for leaving home. Then it was I who was the stranger, and in the various lands I visited I found out at first hand what it is like to be a *peregrine,* a *pellegrino,* or a *pellegrin.* In the fourteenth century the English word for all this activity became, in time for Chaucer's pious and bawdy crew to capture it as their own on their way to Canterbury, simply, *pilgrim.*

People were not any "better" in ancient days than they are now—or, so I believe. Yet we of the twentieth century begin only now very gradually to emerge from a period of intense material-ism during which personal relationships, like our relation to the earth itself, have suffered a devastating loss of richness and of grace. Perhaps we needed to begin running out of material things, and thus to become in some sense primitives again, before we could stop to wonder whether things were really what we wanted most of all. We are tired and confused today about matters as basic as our right to be alive and to inhabit the planet at possible cost of despoiling it altogether. It is an adventure of the heart and a recovery of our own humanity at such a time to read the statutes for care of sick pilgrims by the Knights Hospitallers of the Order of St. John of Jerusalem in the twelfth century A.D.:

How our Lords the Sick Should be Received and Served:

When the sick man shall come . . . let him be carried to bed and there . . . each day before the brethren go to eat, let him be refreshed with food charitably according to the ability of the house.

The beds of the sick should be made as long and as broad as is most convenient for repose, and each bed should be covered with its own coverlet ... and each bed should have its own special sheets ...

Little cradles should be made for the babies of women pilgrims born in the house ...

The Commanders of the houses should serve the sick cheerfully, and should do their duty by them, and serve them without grumbling or complaining ...

Moreover, guarding and watching them day and night ... nine serjeants should be kept at their service, who should wash their feet gently, and change their sheets ...

Throughout the history of the hospice (or of the *hospitium,* "hôtel-Dieu" or "hospitall," for these concepts were for a number of centuries interchangeable) one finds again and again the sense of life itself as a journey, a pilgrimage, and a sojourn among strangers—a "trip" as some now say—toward some future state of rest and blessedness. In a time of reexamination of material values and of renewed spiritual questing, it is no coincidence to find hospices once more appearing on the scene. At the present time in somewhat different guise, aided by every advantage of modern medicine, psychology, and clinical pharmacology, the hospice concentrates its energies upon dying individuals, their families and friends. If they are alone in the world, the hospice community becomes their own.

In England there are some 40 such hospices already in operation. A larger, rapidly increasing number of hospice teams and facilities are now beginning to appear in widespread locations, particularly in Northern Europe and throughout the United States, the best and most advanced of these using as their model of excellence St. Christopher's Hospice in London. Of the modern hospice concept, Dr. Cicely Saunders (founder and director of St. Christopher's) says, "This is indeed a place of meeting. Physical and spiritual, doing and accepting, giving and receiving, all have to be brought together ... The dying need the

community, its help and fellowship . . . The community needs the
dying to make it think of eternal issues and to make it listen. . . .
We are debtors to those who can make us learn such things as to
be gentle and to approach others with true attention and
respect."

The modern hospice: a place of meeting, a way station, a place
of transit, of arrival and departure. And yet, how different from
the airport, the hotel lobby, the hospital. It is the difference in the
quality of human life assumed and provided for, that makes for
the contrast we shall see in the chapters to follow. People in
hospices are not attached to machines, nor are they manipulated
by drips or tubes, or by the administration of drugs that cloud the
mind without relieving pain. Instead, they are given comfort by
methods sometimes rather sophisticated but often amazingly
simple and obvious; and they are helped to live fully in an
atmosphere of lovingkindness and grace until the time has come
for them to die a natural death. It is a basic difference in attitudes
about the meaning and value of human life, and about the
significance of death itself, which we see at work in the place
called *hospice*. The reasons for that difference are worth looking
at, in some detail.

Not Like You and Me

CHAPTER 2

[In sixteenth-century Spain] the sick became the precious possession of the community. . . . The incurably sick had the love of the people and the royal favor, for heaven was open to them.

Dieter Jetter

Each one thought or felt, "Well, he's dead but I'm alive! . . . He has made a mess of things—not like you and me!"

Leo Tolstoy

Will *you* turn me out if I can't get better?

Patient entering
London hospice, 1960s

Green-black against the twilight sky and echoing with birdsong, the pines of Epidaurus still stand, guarding the cool and flowery valley sacred to the healing god *Asklepios*. Here Maria Callas sang *Medea* recently before a wildly cheering audience of 20,000 in an amphitheatre whose aesthetic grace and acoustical perfection have yet to be surpassed. The theatre was built as an integral part of the patient-care system devised by Greek physicians of the fifth century B.C.

The history of medical practice in the Western world is, of course, a subject far beyond the scope of the present study; however, there are a few key spots and a few moments in time worth examining closely in the process of centering down upon the hospice concept. Contrast and comparison are useful in helping us to understand exactly what a hospice is, and what it is not.

Epidaurus was not a hospice. Actually it resembled in many ways one of our vast, modern medical centers today, though it differed somewhat from such places as the Columbia-Presbyterian Hospital in New York or the University of California Medical Center in San Francisco. Modern diagnostic machinery was not available and a great many useful curative procedures had yet to be invented. However, Epidaurus was definitely a place of healing, with a powerful mystique and system of its own. Temples of the most exquisite design stood near the amphitheatre, decorated with the finest carvings of the day and sheltering statuary of ivory and gold. Here also were a superb gymnasium, as well as thoroughly hygienic lavatories, treatment rooms, and baths of the sort one would expect to find now at an elegant spa. The best of contemporary medical treatment was available, including a number of procedures such as hypnotherapy and behavior modification, which are only being rediscovered at the most enlightened of hospitals today, such as the Pain Management Center of the Mayo Clinic, and the City of Hope National Medical Center in Duarte, California.

Twenty-five hundred years ago in the history of the universe as we know it is merely the blink of an eyelid in time. Let us suppose that I have some ailment that has not responded to a day or so in bed with a hot water bottle and a dose of good herb tea. The thing to do, obviously, is to proceed to Epidaurus for my cure. I am a retired soldier, let us say, or a courtesan out of favor this season. I suffer a devastating pain in my lower back, and I arrive feeling dreadful.

I arrive, and am bathed, first in mud-baths, then in steam, and last in fresh tubs of water, first very hot, then tepid, then cool. Now I am gently annointed and massaged with fragrant oils. The attending physician arrives and gives me a carefully programmed regime of physical exercise. In particular, I am urged to take long, quiet walks in the beautiful countryside around us. A sense of well-being and peace begins almost immediately to enter my consciousness and to seep through all my muscles and my nerves.

Next I am questioned about my eating habits and am placed, alas, upon a sensible dietary regime. Hot milk and honey, fruit juices, and water alone it will be for those of us who have been overindulging at the table of late. Others will have fresh vegetables and cheese as well, along with bread, olives, nuts, and other wholesome fare. We are required, as part of our cure, to go to the theatre regularly, there to witness the most hilarious comedies and the most horrifying tragedies of the day. Now we experience *katharsis* of the emotions that have kept our bodies tense, rigid, defended. We laugh, we weep, we scream, we shout. We listen to glorious music by the hour, and we feast our eyes on the beauty of the landscape, the art, the sculpture, and the architecture around us. Thus the healing process begins.

But the best is yet to come; for the greatest curative power to be found at Epidaurus is in a long portico of marble facing the temple of Asklepios and known as the *abaton*. On the open porch of the abaton we lie visited by moon and by wind, by birds and by starlight, not only to rest and to sleep, but most significantly, to dream. Our dreams—even as in the most ancient of Egyptian healing temples and as in the offices of psychoanalysts today—will be interpreted as messages, as ways and means of completing our diagnosis and our cure. Messages from the gods, they were called in those days, rather than messages from the unconscious: a bit more flattering, put that way, and leaving a good deal less doubt as to whether or not they should be acknowledged.

The rate of cure at such a place as Epidaurus was, no doubt, spectacular. The pain in the old warrior's back went away, as such pains are apt to do, without a spinal disc operation. The businessman's ulcer, the migraine of the nervous politician, and the dyspepsia of the *bon vivant* all vanished here in due course. So did the psychosomatic tics and paralyses of the anxious, the vague arthritic aches of the lonely and the bereaved, and the simple boils of the unbathed. Epidaurus was a magnificent medical happening, rather as if in our own time Dr. Freud, Dr. Jung, and Elizabeth Arden had managed to collaborate with Hollywood and HEW in a vast project designed, simply, to make people feel better. Anyone who surrendered to such an environment and who followed such a thoroughly delightful and sensible regime would be certain of improvement; unless, of ourse, he or she were quite hopelessly and incurably ill.

And that, in this particular situation, was Catch-22. The rule at Epidaurus was that people who were hopelessly ill were not admitted. Terminal cases had to go somewhere else to die; and if they had no other place to go, then the field or the side of the road would have to do.

The Greeks were a hardhearted people, of course—not like you and me. On the other hand, any efficient administrator of a medical facility nowadays would be likely to understand the problem. The reputation of the staff—the image of Epidaurus as a place of healing—is at stake. Imagine trying to operate such a place on a pay-as-you-can basis of remuneration from grateful patients—in other words, from patients who have been cured! The overhead is incredible. The local farmers are always overcharging us, the politicians are breathing down our necks. The doctors are making a fuss about conditions, the playwrights are constantly quarreling among themselves, and meantime, the actors steal our drugs. We can't keep an operation such as this going, if people come here and die, and clog up the works. If anything of that sort does manage to happen, we'll simply have to load the body out the back way and hope everyone assumes it happened somewhere else.

Crossing the field now, appearing over the horizon at the most awkward of all possible moments as usual, comes our old friend, the pilgrim. He has come by ship this time, from one of the Aegean Islands, perhaps, or up from Africa. He has walked the long, dusty road up from the port of Naufplion, knowing that he is very ill, but having no coin left in his purse to buy or rent a donkey to carry him. At dusk he arrives, limping, hungry, frightened, and in desperate pain. He has reached the sacred precincts at last. The lamps are being lit beside the holy temple, and the smell of fresh-baked bread is in the air. But our friend the pilgrim unfortunately has a cancer and the hour of his death is now upon him; therefore, he will be turned away.

The classical world differed in many ways from ours. However, they did admire the perfectly formed, beautifully groomed, and healthy human body with as fervent a passion as we in America do today. Men did a great deal of jogging in ancient Greece.

Women of Athens dyed their hair, painted their faces, plucked their eyebrows, and used depilatories. One method commonly used for improving the race was the practice of "exposing" infants who were ill or unattractive and letting them die upon a mountainside; superfluous girl children were also eliminated in this convenient way. Thus the survivors were apt to be healthy as well as handsome, and useful to the state.

Very practical, all this—and yet, one wonders whether these marvelously accomplished people were missing something. It must be admitted that Epidaurus and similar centers of healing throughout the ancient world offered better cures for many common ailments of mankind than are to be found at the average hospital today. And, after the fashion of what is beginning to reappear as "holistic medicine," they treated emotional and physical problems as an integral unit. This, obviously, was an intelligent thing to do. However, the view of the *value* of human life is, per se, here curiously limited, lacking in dimension as if the figures involved turned out, after all, to be cutouts made of cardboard. The ordinary Greek of the day was no Socrates. He believed that he and his fellows were moved about hither and yon from place to place by the mischievous company of gods who pulled the strings, and watched it all from their gallery on Mount Olympus. When the gods were no longer amused, the human beings were simply cast aside. In such a system, a glittering aristocratic superstructure may be maintained, without a second thought, upon a base consisting of the labor of human slaves. In such a world as this, the basic concept of hospice is as yet unborn.

Hospitals there were, in the fully modern sense of the word, only a few centuries later, under the rule of Rome. Interestingly enough, they were constructed for the purpose of mending three classes of people considered particularly useful to the Empire, and therefore too valuable to be cast aside to die: warriors, gladiators, and slaves. In a powerful yet vulnerable military state, the soldier was obviously an important unit. Gladiators were prized after the manner of modern rock stars or professional football players for their entertainment value to the populace; and slaves, even in those days, were apt to be expensive. The Romans were fine, solid builders and great efficiency experts as well. Two thousand years of hospitals following theirs in the Western world have reflected the Roman way of housing the wounded and of organizing their care.

Soldiers, gladiators, slaves. Again, it was a supremely practical way of looking at things. None of these had the power or the means to summon the private physician to his home—if indeed he had anything he could call home. Yet, each was a member of a class judged indispensable to the welfare of the body politic, and thus, if hurt or diseased, must be cured if possible.

One can easily imagine the atmosphere in these *valetudinaria*, as they were called: wooden barracks set on the square with small rooms and symmetrical corridors around four sides, stark and well scrubbed. The model, both architecturally and tactically, was strictly a military one with a highly rational, hierarchical division of labor. In the bare, echoing halls one could hear at all hours of day and night the hurrying feet of the attendants, cleansing wounds, sewing them up; and of others, more highly skilled, setting bones and performing surgery. One would hear the cries of the wounded, the voices begging for water, for wine, for opium; and the consultations of the various caretakers and surgeons among themselves.

The skills of the Roman physician were indeed extraordinary, but it is difficult to find much of anything else to applaud in a place so coldly cynical in its intent. No patient here has control over his own present situation or his own future; he is merely a tool of that society's war against chaos, broken and needing to be mended for other people's convenience. The slave, when mended, takes up his function as a unit of mechanical energy. The soldier is off to battle again, as soon as he is able. And the gladiator with mended wounds goes once more into the arena to provide entertainment for the howling masses. Who, in such a hospital as this, might one day stop and think, *Here lies a human being before me, living, dying, feeling, suffering?* How might any "well" person in such a place even begin to consider the reality of the situation: that the sick individual being "cared for" here is a person with a mind, a heart, and a soul?

Setting these questions aside for the moment, let us turn to a description of the treatment received by a dying patient of our own time, in a large, modern teaching hospital that prides itself upon the excellence of its patient care. The individual in question was the mother of a professor of medicine at one of our Eastern universities, with full access to what we are accustomed to considering the finest of medical expertise:

> What happened was a nightmare of depersonalized institutionalization, of rote management presumably related to science and based on the team approach of subdivision of work. . . . Different nurses wandered in and out of my mother's room each hour, each shift, each day, calling for additional help over a two-way radio. . . . They were trained as part of a team "covering the floor" rather than aiding a sick human being. ... . Laboratory studies of blood and urine continued to be performed, fluids were given, oxygen was bubbled in, antibiotics were administered; the days went by but seemed to be years. The patient was seen occasionally by large groups of physicians making rounds, presumably learning the art of practicing medicine properly. . . . The chart was enlarged regularly with "progress notes." These hastily scrawled writings always dealt with laboratory data, never about the feelings of the patient or her family. . . . One report stated that occult blood had been found in the stool. Someone responded by writing in the chart that, in view of this finding, sigmoidoscopic examination and a barium enema were indicated. I suggested to the author that his conditioned reflexive act was not warranted in the care of an unconscious 80-year-old woman who wanted to die gracefully . . .

Marvelous and, indeed, almost miraculous as the performance of our acute-care systems may be; much as we need and appreciate the heroic efforts of modern physicians to cure us when cure is possible; much as we admire the diagnostic and curative powers of present-day technology when these powers are appropriately used; this is the sort of situation that can only be called intolerable. When the patient's body has become merely an object, a public commodity, and a pawn in our irrational war against death, then it is time to call a halt to such proceedings.

Attorneys, judges, politicians, clergymen, and professors of medical ethics all over the country are struggling as these words are being written, to redefine the circumstances under which one may properly "pull the plug" for patients whose lives in fact have already ended. The moral issues involved are extremely delicate, and it is fitting that they should be studied with great care. Indeed, the questions we are forced to ask one another in this respect may not have any corresponding answers which are always and everywhere and in each possible circumstance, morally right. Still, we must ask them and do the best we can with them; technology now demands this service of us, since we are able to keep people technically alive under conditions which were not dreamed of by those who first set forth to heal the sick. Living wills, euthanasia, and suicide have become, for the same reason, topics of increasingly anxious public concern and discussion of late.

What is not so well known—and even less so in America than in England today—is that we have already available a better model for the care of the terminally ill than any that is to be found, either in the institutional world of classical antiquity or in the conventional medical center of the present time. The ancestor of this model has been available to us, in fact, for nearly two thousand years. While the *valetudinaria* still labored to mend their servants at the borders of the Empire, rather quietly and inconspicuously the first of our modern hospices were born.

Exactly where and when this happened, it is of course impossible to say. Ancient monastic ruins give us hints, and there are other signs in certain heaps of rubble here and there, beside

old village walls. Every now and then some delightful scrap of
written record has a way of turning up, usually in Latin, Spanish,
or French, telling us the rules of such and such an establishment,
or listing the medicines, the loaves of bread, and the jugs of wine
that have been provided during the past twelve months for the
sick. The Hospitaller Knights of St. John of Jerusalem were great
compilers of information about what became, in their case, an
organized network of hospices throughout the civilized world.
However, their flowering was not until the time of the Crusades,
whereas we can hear at least one voice out of history speaking
quite clearly on our subject, at a time many hundreds of years
earlier.

It is the voice of the Roman Emperor Julian the Apostate
speaking in A.D. 361, and essentially he is complaining, not only to
the populace at large, but to himself. The Christians are making
an intolerable nuisance of themselves in Rome. Julian passionately
wants his people to pay proper attention to the gods of their
forefathers, but it is reasonable to assume that military power, as
usual, is the ultimate issue at hand. His borders are overextended,
the German tribes are threatening from the north, and it is
impossible for the Emperor to cope with such a situation while
things are getting more and more difficult at home. They have
tried, over the past few hundred years, feeding these rebellious
people to the lions, burning them alive, and nailing them up by
the thousands in the Colosseum. Nothing, however, seems to
work. More and more of them keep appearing on the scene and
refusing to pay homage to the gods and the authorities or to
behave in any reasonable way whatever.

He asks himself, why do the masses flock to this strange new
faith, knowing full well what the penalties may be? Why is it that
this weak, unruly, and essentially undefended group of individuals
has become a political power that simply must be reckoned with?
The Emperor Julian watches them. They are a queer people,
indeed. They wash the wounds of lepers, and give them food.
They embrace the most utterly useless members of society—the
poor, the orphans, the prisoners, the dying, and the blind. Every
human wreck and stray mendicant in Rome, Christian, Jew,
Pagan, believer or non-believer, is in some mysterious way their

friend. Not only that, but a wealthy Roman matron by the name of Fabiola, evidently turned Christian, has now opened a place of refuge for weary pilgrims. If they are well, she feeds them and houses them and sends them on their way. If they are ill, she nurses them, and if incurably so, she cares for them tenderly until they die. She sees some value in them, evidently.

Why all of this is happening, the Emperor does not quite know; but he is an able politician and he fully understands the danger of it. He issues a proclamation. It is time, he says, for all good pagans to change their ways. Something is stirring in the land that may in the end defeat us, unless we are sensible enough to co-opt its power. "What makes these Christians such powerful enemies of our gods," he says, "is the brotherly love they demonstrate toward the sick and the poor." He urges all Roman citizens immediately to begin imitating them.

In every religion there are saints, and among people of every culture on earth, there have been those who perceived something of holiness or ultimate worth in their fellow human beings. It would be foolish indeed to suggest that Christians invented compassion, or that they alone stand witness to the transcendental dimension of life. However, the coming of Christianity to the center of Western political power does represent a turning point in the moral life of the classical world. From this time on it was no longer possible for a civilized society in the West to ignore the needs of its helpless and afflicted members. The greatest humanitarian movement in the history of the world was now in progress, and with it an expansion of the human consciousness that continues today.

"It was so strange," said a patient entering a London hospice recently, after being discharged from an ordinary hospital. In other places, she explained, "no one seemed to want to look at me." She was dying of cancer, and to look at her might have meant to see, in a place where only successful cure was acceptable, that she was incapable of being cured. To look at her might have meant to see failure, and with it the terror of one's own inescapable death. To look at her, in fact, might have meant, to see *her*.

"The hospice teaches a new attitude," says Leonard M. Liegner, M.D., "with the realization and conscious acceptance of dying and death as part of being born and part of the struggle of life." If the dying patient can be perceived first as a person, and as an individual accomplishing an important part of a full life-cycle, then care givers can concentrate upon giving what is really needed in the situation. They can actively prevent the interference of mindless technological tricks, and can instead provide surcease from physical and emotional pain. They can offer, instead of mechanical resuscitation, a hospitable place in which the personal and spiritual growth of the individual can continue during the process of dying.

In the medieval Christian world, the offer of hospitality to the hopelessly ill and the dying was based on a literal interpretation of the text, "inasmuch as ye have done it unto one of the least of my brethren, ye have done it unto Me." The names of many modern hospices now operating in England give evidence that they, too, are instructed by the New Testament command: St. Joseph's, St. Christopher's, St. Ann's, St. Margaret's, St. Luke's. However, the doors of these hospices are open to persons of every faith and creed, and from any true hospice, no atheist or agnostic will be turned away.

> Oh, let me e'er behold in the afflicted and the suffering, only the human being.
>
> Rabbi Moses ben Maimon

> [When the Chinese came] with the personal—the person put foremost, Ed was no longer "a case." . . . The doctors' tact and tranquility generated ease and there was no feeling of secretiveness or estrangement. A community had formed, and we were an integral part, no longer outsiders waiting in an impersonal corridor for piecemeal information, hesitant to intrude in an area beyond our ken. . . . Our meetings were microcosms of what I had seen and read about Chinese society. . . .
>
> Lois Wheeler Snow

To be with a person who is dying, to share consciousness with him, and to help him die consciously is one of the most exquisite manifestations of the Bodhisattva role.

Baba Ram Dass

Perceptions such as these span the centuries and reach around the globe. In America today the hospice movement appears to take its energies from a more secular, or at least, a more broadly ecumenical base than in the United Kingdom. However, it was a Jewish patient who gave the first £500 toward the founding of St. Christopher's in London, saying to Cicely Saunders at the time, "I want to be a window in your home." While under the care of Dr. Saunders, who is a deeply committed Christian, this young man, who had escaped from the ghettos of the Hitler regime, experienced a rebirth of his faith in Judaism. And this is what the hospice concept is really all about, for this is true "cherysshing"— true hospitality.

Lest Strangers Should Lose Their Way

CHAPTER 3

The truth knocks on the door and you say, "go away, I'm looking for the truth. . . ."

> R. M. Pirsig, *Zen and the Art of Motorcycle Maintenance*

Thus King Stephen gave the Yorkshire manor of Steynton upon Blakhommer ". . . to receive and entertain poor guests and pilgrims there, and to ring and blow the horn every night at dusk lest pilgrims and strangers should lose their way."

> M. R. Clay, *The Medieval Hospital of England*

The healer has to keep striving for . . . the space . . . in which healer and patient can reach out to each other as travelers sharing the same broken human condition.

> Henri J. M. Nouwen, *Reaching Out*

In his immense and gleaming white, air-conditioned cruise ship, the twentieth-century traveler docks at dawn in the port of Rhodes in the Aegean Sea. The "package deal" offered seven islands in eight days, or eight islands—was it?—in ten. By now he is in a state of exhaustion which prevents him from remembering quite how many, or what all the names of them were. He has paid his fare in advance—a good deal more, counting extras, than he could comfortably afford—and yet, despite luxurious food and drink, and blue seas and harbors fulfilling the glossy promise of the brochure, the trip has been, for him thus far at least, curiously unsatisfying. *Too many damn tourists,* he mutters to himself, waiting in line for the narrow approach to the gangplank. *No matter where you go these days, they're always there ahead of you.*

Inching forward in the crowd, clutching his camera and his guide book, he passes a mirror and for a moment fails to recognize himself. He looks again, then takes out his comb and runs it through his thinning hair, worrying about the sunburn beginning to blister on the end of his nose, and about how much to tip the cabin steward at the end of the journey. Trapped in place for the moment, he gazes into his own eyes. Here he is, packed into a swarming mass of people, with his wife nearby and the well loved bodies of his teenaged children pressing close against him; and yet, in some awful way he cannot fathom, he is utterly alone.

Ten minutes later, they are on the dock. A brown-skinned man, half naked and wearing a yellow turban, is pounding a small octopus with rhythmic strokes onto a worn stone block. *Local color.* Older men squat, ignoring the new arrivals, mending yellow nets. *Natives.* Automatically, he stops to take a picture of them.

The traveler looks up at the city of Rhodes. He sees tremendous medieval walls, battlements, towers, banners, gates, and beyond the walls, the tops of cedars and palms, and the graceful minarets of mosques. He is surrounded now by odd, spicy odors and the cries of hawkers from the bazaar, but looking up at the battlements, something else stirs in him like the memory of a dream from long ago, and he shivers, standing in the fierce, sauna-heat of the morning sun.

Hesitantly the traveler moves away from the rest of his family, looking up a street inside the gates, a narrow passage slanting upward, paved with disk-shaped stones set on edge in cement, and sure to hurt his feet. He has worn the wrong shoes for this. "Where are you going?" ask the others. "Well, I don't quite know," he answers humbly—a modern pilgrim without a destination. "I just had a feeling. I'll look for you later, at the ship. I just thought—well—that I'd wander around for a little while." With these words, a vague wave of the hand, and an apologetic smile, he stuffs his guide book into his pocket and sets off alone, up the Street of the Knights, in search of his past.

In the deep shade of early morning, the narrow street is comparatively quiet and cool. Beside him on doorways are the elaborately decorated shields of the various national orders of the Hospitaller Knights of St. John; beyond iron palings he glimpses inner courts filled with blooming oleanders, oranges, geraniums; he sees fountains and hears the sound of plashing water. At the end of a long climb he reaches the *Castella*, but it is not a place of mystery and enchantment as he had rather romantically supposed. It is a brute of a castle, meaning business of another sort— wealth, intelligence, and a tremendous concentration of military power. The rooms above, he finds, are vast and echoing, set about with hulks of carved and gilded furniture, tapestries, urns, mosaics. He feels distinctly uncomfortable here, knowing that it is art, but not being sure whether or not it is the kind of art he is supposed to like.

The order was founded, he is told by the keeper of the *castella*, in Jerusalem in the eleventh century A.D., when some merchants from Amalfi obtained permission from the Caliph of Egypt to build a way station there for sick and weary pilgrims. One Brother Gerard managed the original place, and his band called themselves "The Poor Brethren of the Hospital of St. John." Thereafter the Hospitallers, pressed by the advancing Saracens, moved on to Tyre, thence to Acre, and eventually to the Island of Cyprus. At Cyprus they first became a naval power of sorts, in the process of providing galley-ships for pilgrims to the Holy Land and arming them against the pirates of the day. Year by year, gifts from the wealthy nobles of Europe increased their power. The military order was first recognized by a Papal Bull of 1113, and the knightly brethren who took charge of it during the Crusades were sworn, as was the custom of the day, to vows of poverty, chastity, and obedience.

The guide moves on, telling of the battle in which the Hospitaller Knights stormed Rhodes in 1306, and of how they held it then, heavily fortified, for two full centuries against the weight of the Moslem onslaught, and, incidentally, how they founded here in the meantime one of the finest institutions for the care of the sick and the wounded that the world has ever known.

Pondering the disquieting question of chastity, the middle-aged tourist is moved to look closely at a massive table in one of the upper rooms. The legs of the table, he discovers peering underneath, are carved upward into the forms of voluptuous female busts, so that the knees of those saintly knights—how long ago was it?—must have pressed and rubbed as they sat in conference against them, just so. All of this is very, very strange, he thinks. Fighting and sanctity, jewels and poverty, cannon balls and naked breasts. He looks around him. Well, what next?

An hour or two later, he is even more thoroughly confused. He has wandered about the Old City with the sense that nothing much has changed here for hundreds upon hundreds of years: streets no wider in places than a man is tall, private houses shut tight against the heat and against the swarm of human traffic on the paving stones, shops beside them open wide, people roasting meat an arm's length away, people making sandals, belts, jewelry, bags, sewing shirts. Old men, toothless and grinning, spitting, hawking vegetables. Women, children, cripples selling fruits, pastries, sweets. A man with one arm. Flowers blazing everywhere, the smell of incense and ginger, garlic and dust. Laundry hanging out red and yellow, mustard-gold, personal laundry in the streets. A ragged pair of underdrawers, pale blue, hanging like a flag, and an urchin in a doorway underneath, naked, sucking a half-cucumber. Women sweating, shouting in a language he cannot begin to understand, and the sour smell of baking bread, and the dark eyes of women watching him go by. The intimacy of it staggers him—the richness and the openness of it all to casual view, as if he were moving around all this time in the hallways of a single house where everyone lived together in a seething mass of contradictions and cross-purposes, not minding it—yes, that was it—not minding it at all. *Life,* he thinks. *Everyone here is alive. I am a ghost.*

Sore-footed, tired beyond reason and feeling more than ever

alone, the traveler finds himself standing at last outside what
seems to be a palace, or an art museum. He consults his book. No,
this was the famous hospice-hospital. He goes in. The tumult of
the marketplace is left behind him, and the light falls into the
central courtyard here in such a way that every line in space
around him seems caught in a sudden stillness. The soaring arches
of the infirmary speak to him of an old form, an old order filled
with blessedness and peace. *This is beauty,* he thinks. *I always
forget what it is, until I see it again.* He climbs the steps slowly, on
his aching feet, and sits by an urn filled with fresh mint, and reads.

In the great hall here, "Our Lords the Sick" were received.
They were gently washed and carried to their beds, each with its
own curtain around it, and there they were served by the noble
Knights themselves, who brought them in vessels of solid silver
none but the best and most delicate of foods and drinks such as a
royal prince might desire. The wisest of physicians visited them
daily, diagnosing and prescribing for their ills, and the director of
the hospital himself was ordered twice each day to speak to each
and every patient, giving comfort and encouragement. After the
evening services, "Our Lords the Sick" were entreated by the
priest to join in the great prayer, dating back to Acre in the
twelfth century, in which they made special intercessions to God
for the rest of the world, since heaven was now so directly open to
them: "My Lords the Sick, pray for the peace of heaven, that God
may bring it to earth; pray for the kings and the cardinals, for the
bishops and for the soldiers; pray for the Pope, and pray for all
poor, weary pilgrims who are now lost on land or at sea; and pray
for us who serve you here, that we may all be brought in time to
the great repose."

All personnel here, the traveler reads, were under the oath of
personal poverty, and even the acceptance of gifts from grateful
patients was forbidden. The knights and attendants ate in their
own quarters, far plainer fare; and if they were unkind to patients
or if they neglected their needs in any way, they were put on
bread and water for a week, and whipped. Whipped? Yes,
flogged, twice a week, Wednesdays and Saturdays.

But wait. Here is something equally odd and interesting. "At

the hospital at Rhodes," he reads, "for the first time, patients with
incurable diseases were separated from all others." And where
were they put? In a group of eleven small rooms clustered around
the second-story balcony, which were also reserved for pilgrims
and travelers.

The tourist stands on the balcony, looking in. The little rooms
are quiet and airy, golden-hued, filled with the sweet smell of old
stone. Swallows flit in and out, silently. *Travelers and incurables,*
he thinks. What does that mean? It means something that catches
him at the heart like the sight of beauty, unmistakable when it
suddenly arrives, no matter how long forgotten. *Travelers and
incurables,* he wonders—*Which am I? I am both, I suppose,
always searching for something, I never know quite what. Feeling
always a little foolish, a little out of place with the dreams I can't
name, and the hopes—always wanting to go somewhere, longing
for another place, another time, another chance to figure out the
meaning of it all. There must be a meaning somewhere, in another
language, perhaps, a different way of being, a level of consciousness I can't quite grasp—But it is always there, just around the
corner waiting for me, waiting to receive me, I've sometimes felt.
And now I know how they must have felt, lying here wondering,
waiting to move on, travelers—incurable travelers—living, dying
here in these little rooms, moving on always into the unknown.
Yes, here am I.* He touches the cool stone wall beside him and in
that instant, fully recognizing himself, he puts down the burden of
being a self separate from all others, and with it the pain of his
aloneness.

So the Poor Brethren of St. John must have felt a thousand
years ago in Jerusalem, looking bare-hearted and undefended into
the eyes of the sick and the dying, finding their own spiritual
substance reflected there. The political and military power that
came eventually to surround this primal experience in battlements, and to decorate it with banners and jewels, never
succeeded in destroying or engulfing it entirely, even within the
Order of the Knights themselves. Six hundred years of their
records show a constant struggle within the organization to

maintain the discipline of its origins, despite the acquisition by gift and by conquest of tremendous wealth.

By the time the Knights Hospitallers were driven from their last great outpost on the Island of Malta in 1798, they had such a treasure in silver that Napoleon was able to melt their plates, their goblets, and their artifacts down to 3,449 pounds of bullion; with this, he paid his entire army for his Egyptian campaign. Some two hundred years earlier they had already become a power so awesome that Henry VIII felt obliged to steal most of their English holdings for himself. Their rise from obscurity, from Cyprus to Rhodes and Malta, to Italy, Germany, England, and throughout the West was a stunning event, particularly in view of the fact that it was begun barefoot and in rags, and that the impulse behind it was a perception so simple that it can be shared by a somewhat shy and confused, camera-draped and sunburned tourist from Atlanta or Chicago today.

If the same man—perhaps we ought to call him Smith—were to waken from his reverie in Rhodes and find himself, not on his cruise ship, nor in the great hall of the Hospitaller Knights, but instead, in a small town in fourteenth-century England, he would find it strangely familiar. Having seen Rhodes, having walked through the streets of the Old City, he will immediately recognize a similar quality of life in medieval Devon or Kent. Again, he will move with a swarming crowd through narrow and cobbled streets, seeing people at either side of him making belts, bags, shoes, shirts, measuring out oil for lamps, sharpening tools, roasting nuts and offering them for sale. Their manner of dress is somewhat different, tuned to a cooler climate, of course; the colors about him are not so exotic, and yet the sense of tumbling richness and variety and vibrancy is there. The people are shouting, laughing, sweating, gossiping, haggling at the produce wagons (it is market day) over cabbages, peas, leeks; arguing the merits of fresh eggs, hens, eels, oysters, pullets, partridges, and unfortunately, swans. The price of a swan in the London market in 1338 was three shillings, but you could eat a peacock cheaper if you liked.

John Smith begins to feel more and more uncomfortable. He

has a notion he ought to understand the language, at least. It seems to be English, of a sort. He catches a word here and there, in the flat, nasal accent of the twentieth-century American midwest; but it is all larded through with other sounds (French? German? Latin? Dutch?) that totally confuse him. Being among strangers, not understanding what is happening, he realizes, reminds him of the time he had a heart attack. Someone put him onto a gurney at the hospital, wheeled him down to the end of an empty hallway, and forgot about him. It all came out right in the end, but by that time he was almost too tired and frightened to care.

Stop being a fool, he tells himself firmly, and gets up again. He reaches for his money, points to a keg of barley brew, and tries to indicate, rather loudly, to the owner that he wants to make a purchase. Immediately a curious crowd gathers around him. I guess they don't understand this kind of money, he thinks. Maybe they want coins. He takes out his coins: Greek, Turkish, American. Closer and closer around him people press, talking *about* him to each other, never *to* him. They smell strange and their hands are clammy. Now they start feeling his arms and legs, poking around his belly to see what he is made of, how strong he is. In a minute, he thinks, they are going to take my camera away from me, and they are going to start taking off my clothes. "Let me alone," he shouts at them. "Get off me, for God's sake." He is very weak and dizzy now, and he sinks down on his knees on the cobbled roadbed, very much afraid that he is really going to be sick.

"Pellegrin!" he hears someone say, a woman's voice, ringing and firm. "Be off with you, let be! The holy man, he calls for God! You there, for shame! Take him to the hospice now, let be!" John Smith is lifted up, and carried through the streets. A woman walks beside him, holding his hand. Into a small, stone building they go now, beside the village wall. Gently he is laid onto a pallet made of straw, resting in a bedstead of rough, brown wood. The light falls from a small, high window past a wooden cross on the wall to the dirt floor beside him. He hears the clucking of hens and pigeons, and sees them, walking around, pecking at the dirt inside

the little house. The woman leans over him, covering him with a
blanket made of wool and tucking a soft scrap of sheepskin under
his head. He had thought she must be older—that voice of
command, and the hand holding his so rough and gnarled—but
her face is very young. "Sleep," she says. "You are safe."

He sleeps. When he awakens, she is there. Three other men, he
sees, are lying in beds nearby him, and a child is playing with a bit
of yarn in the sunlight by the door. The man closest to him is very
old, and he moans as if he is in pain. The woman is bathing his
forehead with a damp cloth that smells of roses.

She looks at Smith and sees that he is awake. Without saying
anything, she brings him a small, round loaf of brown bread,
washes his hands and face with the same sweet-smelling cloth,
and indicates that he should eat. The bread has a nutty flavor, rich
and sour. When he has eaten, she hands to him a steaming mug of
something powerful to drink. It resembles wine, or beer, but there
is honey in it too, he thinks, and something else — he cannot tell
what. She watches, evidently with great satisfaction, while he
drains it to the last drop. Then she turns to the old man next to
him, and begins to rub his withered old arms and shoulders, bare
under the blanket, humming something like a nursery song as she
rubs. The old man breathes deeply, and grows quiet.

John Smith realizes that the potion he has drunk was something
very powerful indeed. It had nourishment in it, as well as the
heady quality that makes him feel like rising up to see if there are
any dragons in the neighborhood needing to be slain, or any
maidens needing to be rescued from a dastardly fate. On the other
hand, he thinks, it might be just as pleasant to turn over and sleep
for a week.

"Is this a hospice?" he finally asks.

"Yes," she answers, smiling. "It is."

"Is a hospice something like a hospital?"

"Oh yes, this is a hospital, a hôtel-Dieu. You are right."

"I don't understand," he says, "but you are very good to me. I
don't know that I belong here, however. I am not really sick, you
see. I was only lost for the moment, and a little confused."

"Yes," she says. "I know. You have come on a long journey.
Now you are safe."

"But I am not like that poor old fellow there," says Smith, lowering his voice. "I mean, I can see that he is not long for this world; but I am all right — I am not dying."

"Not dying?" Her smile has a hint of mischief in it now. "Not dying! Well, that is strange, indeed. Were you not born of woman, sir? I was." She turns to the child, and asks her to fetch a pitcher of water and a cup.

"What about the child? What is she doing here? Is she sick?"

"Her parents did not want her. Therefore she belongs to God, and she stays here with me and the other sisters. Now, my dear . . ." For a moment, John Smith thinks she is talking to the little girl, but she is talking to him. She pours a cup of cool water for him and gives it to him, looking with her young-old face and her smiling eyes deep into his own. He takes a sip of the water and wonders what will happen now, as she sits quietly, watching him. Evidently she is ready to sit here peacefully beside him as long as he wants her to stay near, not saying anything or expecting anything of him, simply being there, paying attention to him- without intruding, offering him her presence.

After a little while, he beings to talk. He tells her at first about the sense of fear that came over him in the village, and then about the strangeness of his experience in Rhodes. He tells her about his childhood on a farm in Indiana, and about a number of things that have happened since that never, until this moment of telling them, seemed to hang together in any way, or to make any sense. Scenes and memories form themselves into patterns as he talks all the long afternoon, shapes that really cannot be conveyed in words, but he senses them there, and in the pauses between, the silences becoming longer seem themselves to take a kind of shape; and words and silences together come at last to form a kind of shining whole — his life. It is the first time that he has ever seen these things, these thoughts and hopes and fragments of experience that belong to him, in such a way. After a while, pausing at length, he decides that there is nothing more to say.

"Except," he adds, "that I still don't really know how I came here, and who you are, and what a hospice is." Holding the old man's hands between her own again, she looks around the bare little room, with its stone walls and wooden rafters, its rough cross pegged to the stone, and the pigeons moving about in the sunlight on the earthen floor, and then she smiles once more at him, a smile radiant with affection and merriment and says, "But you do know. Hospice is just this —what you know now, what you see here."

It may be something rather worse than a death-sentence, I am afraid, to send poor John Bunyan Smith III back to vodka martinis, rock music, and Valium on an air-conditioned ·cruise ship after an interlude such as this. Go he must, but perhaps he may be allowed to take with him a prescription from the Franciscan master of medieval pharmacology, Roger Bacon (ca. 1214-1294). If he looks at it from time to time and takes it seriously, he may manage to survive his allotted portion of the twentieth century in reasonably good shape. Brother Roger's own favorite medicine was fresh rhubarb, and his prescription for good health and long life was, "Joyfulness, singing, the sight of human beauty, the touch of young girls, warm aromatic water, the use of spices and strengthening electuaries, and bathing on an empty stomach after getting rid of superfluities."

Superfluities, of course, are what we fill our lives with when we exist in a state of emotional poverty and spiritual starvation. The medieval world we have glimpsed here, in its simplicity and in its splendor, in England and at Rhodes, had a centered and intentional wholeness about it that we do not often allow, or even perceive as a possibility in our own lives. In our society, the child does not play in the corner of the room where the old man is dying, and she is not asked to help with the nursing of the sick. If she is a waif, she is sent to an orphanage; if her parents are wealthy and conscientious, to a boarding school and then, on holidays, to camp. The old person is wheeled to the end of the hall in the general hospital, and there forgotten. Recent studies have shown that nurses take, on the average, twice as long to respond to the call-bell of the dying patient as they do to those of patients who are apparently recovering; and doctors themselves, feeling helpless in the situation, tend to avoid visits to the terminally ill. If the old man has no obvious symptoms requiring immediate treatment, or if he is mentally disabled beyond repair, then he is put away in a home for the aged, out of sight. When we walk down the street, we try not to look at the man who has only one arm; cripples are invisible to us. Our own wounded condition as ordinary human creatures living in the midst of a mystery we cannot fathom, yearning for something better, becomes a matter of shame to us, like a set of ragged underwear that must at all costs be concealed. In the process of thinking this way we ourselves become partially invisible to ourselves, partially lobotomized, so that we walk the streets of our own cities like ghosts and trespassers, feeling — as indeed we often are — a little less than human.

It would be a mistake to return to all known procedures of medieval medical care, of course. In all probability the village we have just visited in England was about to be ravaged by bubonic plague, which carried away one-fourth to one-third of the population of Europe in the fourteenth century, and which now can be cured by a simple course of antibiotics. We now know about germs, and we know that the young hospice-keeper (who was a lay sister of the local priory, trained and skilled only in the simplest nursing procedures of the day) should not have used the same perfumed cloth to wash the hands of John Smith that she had used to wipe the spittle from the face of the dying old man. These are good and useful things to know, for we cannot hope to improve the quality of life without paying attention, in the meantime, to appropriate ways and means of preserving life itself.

Still, we may learn an important lesson in humanity from the great hospice-hospital in Rhodes, and from the simple hostel for the sick and weary in our nameless English village. From Turmanin in Syria, St. Gall's in Switzerland, from the Hospice de Beaune in France and from the hundreds upon hundreds of way-stations established on similar principles in medieval days, we of the twentieth century can take renewal and refreshment. Such places of welcome remind us with great force and power that we are all one family, all seekers and wanderers on the face of the earth. They also help us to remember that what happens to the mind and the spirit at any given time is at least as important as what happens to the body. *L'hygiène physique et morale des malades* (the physical and moral hygiene of the sick) was attended to at Beaune, where a treasure of art and architecture and a fine library, as well as clean linen and wholesome food, were provided for the ill and the dying. Monastic attendants throughout Europe in the Middle Ages not only heard confessions and offered spiritual comfort to sufferers, but gave them fellowship in the acknowledgment of our common, broken, and imperfect human condition. The dying were seen as individuals useful to mankind, not in terms of what organs they might contribute to those living after them, or as objects of scientific speculation, but as beings moving forward, more rapidly than others, on the metaphysical plane.

At the farthest frontiers of modern science, physics now begins to meet again something that can only be called metaphysical. Moving beyond the structural limitations of medieval thought, we find evidence at quite another level of the permanence of energy, and of the insubstantiality of matter. Less and less it becomes possible for us to state that the medieval view of dying as a form of transformation was wrong. In taking the name *hospice* for a newly intelligent and compassionate mode of caring for the dying, we reconfirm what was best in the vigor—both physical and spiritual—of village life in other times.

Nothing that is human is excluded from the premises, or from the consciousness, of hospice life. Beauty here is not a matter of tidy appearances, logical proprieties, or even of physical prowess. Rather, it pertains to those exchanges between people, living and dying, who value one another as vessels of a purer and more lasting force — who look beyond present turmoil and incapacity, to the realization that our entire planet has now become one village seeking to be healed. With the spread of the hospice concept in our culture, many of us may discover that we are learning from the sick how to be well again, and from the dying, how to live.

Doing It

CHAPTER 4

The First Law: Do it! Money will come when you are doing the right thing.

Michael Phillips *The Seven Laws of Money*

. . .While we look not at the things which are seen, but at the things which are not seen: for the things which are seen are temporal; but the things which are not seen are eternal.

II Corinthians 4:18

November 11, 1976, Marin County, California, a few miles north across the Golden Gate from San Francisco. After the long drought of summer, a cold gray rain is falling steadily. At 7:00 A.M. it is still quite dark, but in the small town of Belvedere, St. Stephen's Episcopal Church presents a parking problem even at this hour. Like a medieval village under one roof, this is a place of widely varied communal activity; the church bulletin mentions not only frequent services here throughout the week, but workshops and seminars in everything, it seems, from dance, hatha yoga, and printmaking to the theology of Dante, Thomas Merton, and Kierkegaard. On the kiosk in the courtyard, I note an invitation to the men of the parish to come on Saturday morning and learn to make bread.

A fire is blazing today in a Franklin stove in the small redwood room adjacent to the parish hall. In the vestibule, the fragrance of good food and coffee mingles with that of wet raincoats and overshoes. Members of the board of Hospice of Marin are arriving for a discussion-breakfast.

Marin's hospice came into being late in November of 1975 when a small group of individuals made the decision to offer their professional services free of charge to dying members of the community and their families. The existence of the modern English hospices was not unknown to them. They were familiar with the work of Dr. Elisabeth Kübler-Ross, and had taken note of the home-care program operated by Hospice, Inc. in New Haven, Connecticut. However, it was out of personal experience and in response to the needs of friends and neighbors that this small, nonprofit corporation was quietly founded.

Since 1975, because such needs within the community have long existed and now are at last beginning to be met, the original group of four has doubled and twice again redoubled its number of volunteer workers, board, and staff. Standards of care have proved not merely acceptable, but enlightening and a welcome boon to the local medical establishment. Public notice now begins to focus upon Hospice of Marin with an eagerness that threatens the young organization with a serious identity crisis. The meeting this morning, in fact, represents a turning point which may be typical in the life of any group which sets out to offer the public with open hands something that it very urgently needs.

The small room begins gradually to be filled with quiet laughter and conversation. Father John Thornton, rector of the church, is also president pro tem of Hospice. Grave and correct in his clerical garb plus a red canvas apron and hiking boots, he serves coffee from a pewter pitcher in front of the fire, welcoming each new arrival with a penetrating glance deep into the eyes, and a quick, warm smile. An instructor of advanced nursing is here from the State University south of San Francisco, and now a gentle, bearded young doctoral student of medical anthropology comes in from the University of California campus in Berkeley across the bay. Both must have risen long before dawn and driven an hour or more in the dark and the rain in order to be here. The president-elect of the County Medical Society hurries in, a distinguished internist who must leave the meeting early to attend to his own practice. The Director of the Department of Aging of the State of California is here, and a San Francisco attorney known to have a good head for business, and also for medieval studies, Tibetan lore, and classical Greek. He stands chatting with a charming lady in proper tweeds, noted locally for her somewhat miraculous skills at fund raising, while the executive director of Hospice of Marin, weary from a recent bout with major surgery herself, pulls up a cushion to sit before the fire.

At 7:30 the state senator of the district comes loping up the path, casually elegant in regimental tie and rumpled rain-gear. Humanitarian, conservationist, and raconteur par excellence, he is the newest member of the board; he has spent many hours recently, nursing his own brother through terminal cancer. The room is filled now, nearly to its manageable limits. The door is closed, but is almost immediately opened again to admit an explosion of human energy, blue-eyed, Viking-sized. Despite armloads of notebooks, the new arrival somehow manages to envelop each person present in his immense and exuberant embrace before settling down to the solemn duties of breakfast. This is William M. Lamers, Jr., M.D.—psychiatrist, writer, lecturer, inventor, fisherman, fisher of men, and philosopher—in whose fertile brain Hospice of Marin was conceived, and who now serves as its Medical Director.

The conversation at breakfast is noisy and full of enthusiasm. I am here as a guest, saying little, listening a great deal, and am aware of being in a sort of time warp just now that includes much that is unseen. Two days ago I was a pilgrim in fourteenth-century England, lying in a little hospice beside a medieval priory. Last night I pored over the ground plan of the magnificent ninth-century monastery of St. Gall's in Switzerland, noting with delight the "Hospice For Pilgrims and Paupers" tucked in beside the "Brewer's Granary" and the "House for Horses and Oxens and Their Keepers." Yesterday a letter came to me from a friend in Geneva with pictures of the Hospice of Saint Bernard, which after eight centuries is still functioning, sheltering travelers and wayfarers of every sort, and rescuing victims of avalanches at the heights of the alpine passes. My head is physically connected with my body, as far as I can tell at this hour of the day, but I realize that it is filled, not only with facts and figures about Hospice of Marin, but with the music and the snows of other ages: with odd scraps of chivalry, banners and bandages, homespun and barley

brew, swans, the laundry hanging in the cobbled streets of
Rhodes, and the shields of the Knights Hospitallers.

The history of hospitals is one thing, I have come to understand, and that of hospices has been, in the past few centuries,
quite another. Since the closing of the monasteries during the
Reformation, the two concepts have split away from one another
and have become separate, and until recently, the hospice process
has gone underground. The St. Bernard dog with the keg of
brandy under his chin now figures in cartoons and comic strips—
familiar enough, but unless one is actually up there shivering in
the snow, rather a joke. Governments and corporations have
assumed the function, which was once purely personal and
religious, of caring for the sick. Scientists have been busy
discovering germs and naming diseases, while medicine itself has
become entangled in a bureaucratic procedure demanding so
much paper work of most physicians that the time and energy
they can give to patients is sorely limited. In 1973, my sources
say, the United States spent 15 percent more on personal and
public health services than on national defense. Of this $94
billion, only 4.2 percent was provided by private philanthropy.
With $140 billion currently budgeted for health, 40 percent will
be spent on hospital care.

Looking around me in the little room, I think of money, which
is tangible and material—and of human energy, which is not.
Hospice of Marin has happened simply because a certain number
of people in a rather unusual, though small, California county felt
that it was the right thing to do. History, in fact, has come full
circle here. Once again we are in the place of original *hospitality*,
where people are willing to labor unrewarded, to see that their
neighbors do not die without grace, and that the families of the
dead do not mourn uncomforted. I realize that I am in the
presence here of an existential force as powerful, and yet as
invisible, as electricity.

What is the source of this energy? I could not presume to speak
for each member of Hospice of Marin, but I do sense that the
source, whether perceived as religious or felt as simply humanitarian, is something partaking of that realm which is eternal, and
abides. Because of the nature of what is being done here, these

people, board and staff and volunteers, are immediately related to a great family of individuals whom they may never meet. I think of Fabiola, who opened her home to sick and weary pilgrims in Rome in the fourth century A.D., and of Jerusalem's Poor Brethren of St. John, and of the nurses of the Hôtel-Dieu in Paris who knelt by the icy banks of the Seine in the eighteenth century washing sheets, without soap.

The problem under discussion today is a crucial one. Hospice of Marin has begun modestly, pooling the skills of its members in medicine, pharmacology, nursing, counseling, psychiatry; learning from St. Christopher's Hospice in London, sharing information with Hospice, Inc. in New Haven, with the Palliative Care Service of the Royal Victoria Hospital in Montreal, with the hospice team at St. Luke's in New York, and others. In the process of development it has deliberately avoided publicity, fearing premature expansion of its commitment to the community at large.

Now the word is out. Small amounts of money have been arriving in the form of donations and grants. At the same time, the number of physicians, patients, and families requesting Hospice aid has suddenly doubled, then tripled. Approximately 600 people die of cancer in the county each year. A few months ago, Hospice of Marin was caring for only four or six patients at one time. Now there are 18, and only yesterday three more urgent calls were received. Some of these patients will require intensive, personal nursing care by Hospice-trained specialists. All must have expert medical and pharmacological supervision. Most will need counseling with therapists, phychiatrists and/or members of the clergy, not only for themselves, but for their nearest of kin. Meantime, people from Hospice stand by the families of those who have already died, offering continued fellowship and support as needed. Somehow all of this must be managed, and managed right. It is inconceivable to the people here that anyone who comes for help to Hospice of Marin should be turned away. The only restriction that, at present, is tolerable is the concentration upon cancer, simply because this is the area of greatest need, and the disease most dreaded.

How then to organize properly, without losing touch with the *esprit* that has already developed? The spirit is strong—stronger than ever, now that Hospice of Marin has shown what it can do. But the flesh is weary, and local banks have a way of reminding people rather regularly when their accounts are overdrawn. Obviously a core group of workers must be put on salary, in order to free them from other responsibilities. No one here really wants to talk about money, but under the circumstances, money in quantity has become a necessity.

One of the ironies of the situation is that in the material sense, Hospice of Marin does not exist at all. It does not own so much as a hut of stone or a bed to put a patient in. *Hospitality*, in this case, is simply wherever the patient is. The state has certified Hospice of Marin as a Home Care Agency, and this will definitely help. Medicare has certified Hospice of Marin for reimbursement; however, they are not yet seeking these funds, pending development of contracts with all medical insurance carriers. The office now runs on small donations, mostly from grateful friends and families of Hospice patients. Two modest grants, which were acceptable because congruent with the true nature and purpose of the work, have been received, and the news now is that a larger grant, equally appropriate, is a distinct possibility.

A distinct possibility, someone remarks, is very nice, but it is not a horse. True enough, it is agreed — not a horse, nor even a unicorn. Nevertheless, enthusiastic plans are made for parceling out this excellent and ethereal animal when it arrives. Simultaneously, it seems, the creature is going to be ridden, raced, put into harness, and caused to pull a wagon; it is also going to provide steaks and soup for the entire staff before getting up to race again; and from there, no doubt, it will be let out at stud. The discussion rambles on until Father Thornton quietly interrupts with a motion, seconded and passed, of a compromise sort. This is a group quite obviously dissatisfied with compromise. In fact, Senator Peter Behr remarks wryly that the whole situation rather reminds him of the man who rushed to the river and tested the depth of the water with both feet at once.

There is a restlessness in the air, as an attempt is now made to redefine the proper relationship between staff and board, and to chart the course of the future in view of rapidly multiplying commitments. The young doctoral candidate voices it: "Until now, Hospice has been a family group, a close community. After a while, if this sort of expansion goes on, I am afraid we will become just one more cold, impersonal institution. I don't like it. I don't feel good about it at all. But what can we do?"

It is a proper question and indeed a challenge for any group of this sort when such a moment arrives. From the records of the Hospitaller Knights to the progess reports of St. Christopher's Hospice in London today, one can see again and again the eternal struggle to combine efficiency with grace, financial sense with intimacy. Perhaps we must simply accept the fact that the tension between the individual and the institution, like the tension between flesh and spirit, or the tension between lovers, is a human constant, part of the very ground of our being. We do the best we can with it, and that is all we can do.

The meeting has ended. We stand now in front of the church, watching red and yellow leaves stream past toward the storm drain at the bottom of the hill. During their brief passage they give off their own light, it seems, into the gloom of the day. The human condition: there it is, and the mystery, that a charged field of energy should transform itself, just so, into the material and the temporal mode. Nothing in the universe is ever really wasted, I believe. And yet it becomes very important for me, just at this moment, to stand in the rain looking at red and yellow leaves.

The following day I have an appointment with Dr. Lamers to discuss the beginnings of Hospice of Marin, and to learn more details about its methods of patient care. Again we meet in front of a blazing fire, this time at his home some 25 miles north of San Francisco. In a booklined room filled with plants of every description, with the largest dining table I have seen since I visited the castle of the Hospitaller Knights at Rhodes, we sit on enormous floor cushions and talk.

In a way, he tells me, it all began with a man named Ed. He goes into his study and brings me a picture of a handsome middle-aged man standing at the edge of a dock or a boat with the water behind him, smiling, not knowing—because no one knew that day—that he was dying of cancer. "Ed was a friend of mine," Dr. Lamers says. "He told me that he wanted to die at home, and so that is what happened. I didn't know then all I now know about medication, but I was sure that he would be more comfortable in an atmosphere of good, loving care and support. Ed had a large family—wonderful people—and I worked with every one of them. We dealt with the realities of it, day by day. And they all came through it beautifully, even the youngest boy, who felt so gypped compared to the others, that he would never have a chance to know his father while he was growing up. I still keep in touch with them, of course. That was ten years ago."

Other families in the community began calling upon Dr. Lamers, after this, to help in similar situations. Colleagues, too, turned to him more and more often for aid with the emotional difficulties of terminally ill patients and their families. He responded by giving his time, evenings, weekends, whatever he could spare from his regular practice of psychiatry. Meantime, his own sister died very suddenly, leaving six young children. Dr. Lamers went immediately to work with them, helping them to comprehend the reality of the situation and involving them as responsible members of the mourning process. He felt that it was important for them to see their mother dead, and to have a chance to say their own goodbyes to her. When the youngest could not reach high enough to look into the coffin and asked to be lifted up, Dr. Lamers did this for him, allowed him to touch her face, and answered his questions truthfully and matter-of-factly, about why her skin felt different now, and why she lay so still.

By the late 1960s, he says, he was exploring the idea of setting up, with some other physicians, a "Center For the Reaction to Loss." He had found in his practice that more than 60 percent of his patients had emotional difficulties directly related to experiences of bereavement or abandonment. These situations had not been freely acknowledged or worked through creatively at the time, and were often buried deep in the unconscious. By now, he was lecturing throughout the country on grief and mourning, the cyclical stages he had observed, first of denial, then of anger and despondency; and finally, in healthy cases, a healing stage bringing with it recommitment to life and the courage to love again. If only, he felt, these processes could be brought to the consciousness of grieving individuals *during the experience itself*, then they might not turn up in psychiatrists' offices 15 or 20, even 30 years later, with lives essentially crippled by unfinished emotional work.

In the course of his lectures, Dr. Lamers often crossed paths with Dr. Elisabeth Kübler-Ross, who was speaking to many of the same audiences about death and dying. Dr. Kübler-Ross, by now a figure of considerable international renown, had noted in her own patients similar cyclical stages of reaction to the prospect of death, and sought to emphasize creative potentials for personal growth in the lives of the terminally ill. It was not until the spring of 1974 in Ogden, Utah, however, that the two met and talked together for the first time. After sharing a platform at Weber State College for a lively question and answer session on their mutual concerns, they met again at a small dinner party and continued their discussions. The following day, Dr. Kübler-Ross confided a wistful ambition: she felt a great and powerful desire, she said, to ride horseback across the great plains above the city and into the Wasatch Mountains. It was impossible that she should ever do such a thing, of course. Since the publication of her best-selling books, she had become completely overwhelmed with the demands of her correspondence, her lecture schedules, and continuing research, while responding to the needs of her own patients as well. And yet, here in the American West, a sense of some spiritual connection with Indian life and lore was so powerful in her consciousness that she longed to free herself, somehow, for such an adventure.

Obviously, Dr. William M. Lamers is the man to see about a horse. One quick phone call and mounts of the flesh-and-blood variety were saddled and waiting. Up toward the mountains they rode at dusk, in a sharp, cold wind with rain clouds hovering. While he struggled with his own large and rather unruly stallion, Elisabeth Kübler-Ross suddenly took off at breakneck pace. "I will never forget that scene," says Dr. Lamers. "It was incredible. She is such a tiny little thing, her feet wouldn't even reach the stirrups, and there she was riding like a demon straight across that wild, enormous space with the dark mountains looming above and the wind blowing, and it was beginning to rain. I was terrified. I thought she was going to fall off and break her neck. She was completely unafraid, having the time of her life. Finally she came back absolutely beaming and said, 'Thank you, that was marvelous.' On the way back she was very quiet—it must have been very hard on her, all that way downhill, though she never spoke a word of complaint—and then suddenly she said to me, 'Bill, I think you should start a hospice in Marin.' "

Hospice? At that point, Dr. Lamers says, he was not even sure exactly what a hospice was. "I had been so busy doing what I was doing all that time, I had never stopped to find out." In 1973, he had been invited to hear Dr. Cicely Saunders speak at Grace Cathedral in San Francisco, but had not been able to attend because he himself was lecturing somewhere out of town that day. "I began to do research on it then, wrote to St. Christopher's, read all of their material, and held extensive discussions with Dr. Arthur Lipman of Yale. Lipman gave me a great deal of helpful information, particularly about the system of medication he had developed with the hospice team in New Haven. John Thornton and I talked about it—he has always been deeply involved, of course, in parish counseling and in his ministry to the sick and the dying—and then in the autumn of 1975, four of us sat down together. John Thornton, Barbara Hill (who is now our executive director), Julie Bloomfield (executive director of the Babcock Memorial Endowment), and myself. We decided to incorporate, and get on with it."

Several important tasks immediately confronted the original Hospice team. First, they had to identify and adopt a fully effective system of pain control. Hospice policy demands that the terminally ill must be kept comfortable and alert—in their own homes, if they wish to be there—and this is a problem which has not, in general, been solved satisfactorily by the medical and surgical establishment. Second, the community had to be informed, even before Hospice of Marin would begin its formal operation, as to exactly what a hospice program can do. There must be no mystery or sensationalism about it; standards of patient care must be legally and medically correct, appropriate, and clearly understood by everyone involved. Special training of volunteer nurses and therapists was the next priority, and only then would come the beginning of full-fledged hospice care.

The following year was a time of education for the growing Hospice of Marin team and for the larger community as well. Fortunately, Dr. Lamers' background in clinical pharmacology is extensive. He did two years of research in the field while at medical school at Marquette University, and during his residency visited the Federal Narcotics Hospital in Lexington, Kentucky. Together with Dr. Frederick Myers, professor of Pharmacology at the University of California Medical Center, he had set up a notably successful program of non-narcotic withdrawal from drug addiction. He had directed and helped to found several well-known local programs in problems of drug abuse; thus he was in a good position, not only to set up the medication program for Hospice of Marin, but to do the work of explaining it to local physicians, pharmacologists, nurses, hospital administrators, and the general public.

One problem for American hospices modeling themselves after St. Christopher's in London is that British law differs from the American in allowing medically supervised use of drugs such as diamorphine (heroin) and cocaine. At St. Christopher's in 1975 an oral medication known as Brompton's Mixture was providing a spectacular degree of relief from pain and distress for terminal cancer patients. It consisted of

Diamorphine HCl	5-10 mg
Cocaine	10 mg
Alcohol (90%)	1.25 ml
Syrup	2.5 ml
Chloroform water to	10 ml

given with a phenothiazine to potentiate the effect of the diamorphine, and to act as an antiemetic and tranquilizer.

However, legally acceptable variations of this prescription

have been developed in America, and at Hospice of Marin a modified Brompton's Mix known as "Hospice Mix" is now proving, according to Dr. Lamers, "amazingly effective." It consists of morphine, alcohol, and usually one of the phenothiazines (Thorazine, Phenergan, Compazine) in a water solution with cherry syrup to partially offset the bitter taste of the narcotic. Initially as much as 10-30 ml of this mixture may be given every 3 or 4 hours; far less becomes necessary as soon as pain is under control, but it is of utmost importance that every prescribed dose be taken, round the clock, night and day. This is done to prevent pain from having the opportunity to build up again. It is also important in Dr. Lamer's system of medication that the patients themselves dispense and administer their own medicine and keep their own "pain charts." In a very short time, under Hospice care, this becomes known as the "comfort chart," and throughout the process, it gives the patient a realistic sense of control over the situation.

Pain control, it turns out, is not so much a matter of what is in the medicine, as it is of how and when it is administered. In a short-term, accident, or acute-care situation, analgesics such as codeine tablets or morphine injections as needed (PRN) may be entirely appropriate. However, terminal care, when severe and chronic pain is involved, presents an entirely different set of demands. Morphine shots and heavy doses of tranquilizers, administered in a clockwork pattern in an automatic and impersonal atmosphere, tend to make screaming addicts or deeply depressed or helpless "vegetable" cases out of dying people who, with the right kind of care and medication, might otherwise be quite serene, clear-headed, and comfortable. The fear of pain increases pain itself by geometric proportions. When severe pain is experienced and is expected to continue indefinitely, even to get worse, the patient enters into a world of horror and hopelessness that for many treated by conventional methods ends only with death. *This is not necessary, and with hospice care it simply does not happen.* Knowing that it is not going to happen is, in itself, part of the comfort offered to hospice patients and their families.

Severe pain is, of course, not always present in cases of terminal cancer. However, other sorts and degrees of physical discomfort are all too apt to appear, such as nausea, vomiting, muscle spasms, headaches, difficulties with bladder or bowel function, anorexia, and other problems which may or may not even be directly related to the presence of the disease. Hospice of Marin personnel are trained to consider seriously and to cope creatively with all such symptoms. Sometimes rather sophisticated medications are necessary, and the literature on these methodologies grows very rapidly of late, on both sides of the Atlantic. At other times, however, procedures for relief of distress can be rather surprisingly simple. Gentle massage, a soft pillow placed just so, a subtle change in diet, a tempting drink, or time taken simply to be present, quietly caring and listening, recognizing the person as a unique and valued individual—these things can truly heal the dying, even when cure has become impossible.

"How do you decide when a patient has come to the point of needing hospice care, rather than active treatment of the disease?" I ask.

"Most of our referrals thus far have been from physicians themselves. If there is any element of doubt, of course we can always ask for an additional opinion. We only work in situations where an attending physician is directly involved. Our work is comfort control, patient and family education and support, total hospice care during the dying process itself, and bereavement counseling. In some cases, we ourselves have recommended further intervention, such as chemotherapy. We have cared for patients who were having chemotherapy at the time, and suffering from the side effects of that. The changes in appearance, loss of hair, and so forth are often very distressing to patients and to members of the family. Our therapists have been able to help people to recognize and to manage the feelings they are having, not only about death and loss, but about the difficulties experienced during the course of illness and treatment."

"This is all very different, then, from the work of an ordinary nursing or convalescent home?"

"Yes, and except for bereavement counseling, which may

continue for some time, it is a comparatively short-term operation as well. We come in where there is a limited life expectancy, usually no more than several months."

"Do people sometimes not want to know or admit that they are dying?"

"They know. We don't press the issue. We try to work with whatever they are able to encompass at the time. In some situations, the family enters into a conspiracy to pretend it isn't so. But we are certain, and there are statistics to prove it, that this kind of deceptive attitude causes serious difficulties in the lives of everyone involved. We work very hard, in such an event, to help the entire family unit face the truth together."

"How do the local hospitals feel about Hospice of Marin?"

"We have their complete support. And this is because we didn't rush into it. We took the time, hour after hour, month after month, to go around and talk with all of them, and to let them know exactly what we were going to do, and why. Let me tell you one story. When we were just beginning to work as a team with patients, less than a year ago it was, I was called in to one of the local hospitals by a physician. He had a woman there with cancer who had become completely unmanageable. She was heavily sedated, crying out hour after hour, and disrupting others on the ward. No one had any idea what to do for her. When I walked into her room, she was curled up in a fetal position, hallucinating, reaching around in the air for things that weren't there. I changed her entire medication system immediately, and as soon as she cleared up a little, began trying to get in touch with what was happening in her head. On the second day, quite free from pain, she sat up, looked me straight in the eye and said to me perfectly calmly, 'I don't want to be here. I know that am dying. I want to go home.' So we enabled her to go home, and in a short time, she died there very peacefully."

"Have you met situations where the family, even with help from Hospice, is simply unable to cope? I am wondering specifically whether you see a need at the present time for a special Hospice building, an inpatient facility?"

"Yes, we would like to have a small freestanding unit with

several beds for certain kinds of circumstances. Sometimes the medical and nursing problems can become temporarily rather acute. Or a family may be in need of a rest from the situation. As it is, we go into the nursing homes and the hospitals and do what we can, but the dying have the right to a great many things that such institutions simply cannot provide. They need life around them, spiritual and emotional comfort and support of every sort. They need 'unsanitary' things, like a favorite dog lying on the foot of the bed. They need their own clothes, their own pictures, music, food, surroundings that are familiar to them, people they know and love, people they can trust to care about them. Hospices can provide this, in their inpatient units; and yet, for many individuals and their families, it is much better for it to happen at home."

I have heard by now of some rather extraordinary instances of personal and spiritual growth among dying people who have received hospice care, both in Britain and in America; before the interview ends, I ask Dr. Lamers to comment on this. The process of dying, as he approaches it, is clearly something to be looked at, felt, admitted, shared, and fully brought into the scope of conscious human activity. *Ars Moriendi,* as it was called in the medieval Christian text, and I am reminded also of the ancient *Tibetan Book of the Dead:* not a book about ghosts, but about how to die consciously, in a state of spiritual enlightenment. Hospice of Marin evidently offers its patients this opportunity, and I wish to know more about how people are responding to it.

The story Dr. Lamers tells me in reply is one of a young boy, fourteen years old, who was suffering from leukemia. When Hospice of Marin was called in, the situation was a desperate one. The boy was at home after extensive treatment which had won him some time without being able to effect a cure. He was very feeble and utterly withdrawn, hostile to a degree that had alienated him entirely from family and friends. The family situation was one of chaos and utmost misery. His mother, in fact, had suffered from depression because of the strain, and was currently in a local hospital. For months previously, she had not been able to communicate with her son, and he had not been willing to speak to her, or even to look at her.

The Hospice team came in. Therapists worked with all members of the family, hearing their feelings and helping them with their immediate, practical difficulties. Dr. Lamers worked with the mother, giving her the psychological support she needed in order to come to grips with reality. Soon she was home again, working beautifully with her own grief, caring for her family, learning to accept help from concerned and loving neighbors, and beginning at last to open up communication with her son. The boy, in turn, sensing the new strengths around him, was able to move out of hiding. The anger and the shame, the misery and the disappointment he had experienced throughout his illness had prevented him from being able to give or to receive love.

The last weeks of his life were made physically comfortable for him; but even more significant was the adult commitment he was finally able to make to those who cared for him. If the quality and not the quantity of life is important, then this boy achieved more than many an octogenarian; and if death at any age can be beautiful, this one was. On the day of his death, when his mother came into his room in the morning, the young boy spoke his last words. She asked him what he wanted for breakfast, and his reply was, "A kiss."

Night Flight

CHAPTER 5

In the Vulgate, [the Greek word for "love"] is sometimes rendered by *dilectio* (noun of action f. *diligere,* to esteem highly, love,) but most frequently by *caritas,* "dearness, love founded on esteem."

Oxford English Dictionary

Describing hospital procedure during the period from the sixteenth century almost to the twentieth century requires a strong stomach.

Mary Risley, *House of Healing*

"This is your captain speaking. We apologize for the delay, ladies and gentlemen," says the voice on the ever-so-slightly faulty loudspeaker system, while the overhead lights blink off and on. "We have had a bit of trouble with our electrical wiring, but that is now mended. The reason for continued delay at present is that we are very heavily loaded tonight, and we must wait our turn for the longest of the jet runways. Relax, please. Make yourselves comfortable. Do not leave your seats. No smoking. Keep your seats in the fully upright position, and keep all seatbelts securely fastened."

The lights now go off entirely. Silence. Dark. The frail, white-haired stranger sitting beside me sighs quietly, clears his throat, and coughs. Something like a deeper sigh stirs in the heavy air around us, but no one speaks. Four seats abreast down the center of the aircraft, plus two or three on either side, times twenty, thirty—how many rows? Three hundred bodies at the least, pressed together arm and shoulder, elbow, knee, and thigh, each sensing the thickness and the heat of the other's substance, breathing in the invisible droplets of each other's sweat, the garlic, mint, and whiskey of one another's breath. Footsteps, running. A door ahead, opening into a half light, closing.

The old man beside me coughs again. His chest rattles. Is he ill? Is he dying, perhaps? Are we all about to die? *Illness creates dependency,* say the sociologists. Illness—well, yes. Being strapped down in such a spot as this creates dependency too. One hundred years ago (have we forgotten it so soon?) English-speaking people on both sides of the Atlantic called their sick *the impotents,* strapped them down in madhouses if they were strange, gave parties to come and laugh at them through the bars while they screamed, locked them up, if they were poor and sick, in workhouses, 50,000 of them at a time in the city of London alone. At Bellevue Hospital in New York, in April of 1860, rats ate the nose, the upper lip, and half of the left foot of a newborn infant. The young mother, lying alongside in the same bed, was too ill and weak to prevent it; she was a charity case. What is *charity?*

The lights come on again now, steady and full. Music plays loudly, a cheerful Strauss waltz. The plane begins to move. We all smile at one another a little sheepishly. Such things—such things as we were thinking about a moment ago—do not happen to us. They happen only to people who are poor and sick, or in another country long ago. The engines roar and the plane plunges down the runway; we laugh and chatter, powerful again, healthy and strong. Soon we will be on our way to London, drinking gin and eating steak. There isn't a person on the plane at this moment who does not believe that he or she is going to live forever.

And yet the runway is long, longer than any runway has a right to be. We are nightmare-heavy, far too slow, it seems, ever to get off the ground. There must be some mistake. We are wallowing along, wings shuddering, everything swaying, lights blinking off and on and off again, broken. Again and again the lifting moment fails us—will there be fire?—then suddenly we are up, we have mastery of it, the corridor to freedom, safety, space, and air.

What gods we are now, what power we have! Nothing can touch us. We are safe. It is we who are still now; earth swings away from us. Furthermore, like gods we now own time: nine hours of it, belonging to us alone. The people we left behind us are part of yesterday—too bad for them—and the ones we are going to see will not be real until tomorrow. The elderly gentleman beside me pats his lips gently with a clean, folded, white linen handkerchief and orders sherry. Cities and towns lie sprawled below us, but their business is none of ours. Distance it is that does it. However, you must be sure not to look down. If you do, and actually believe what you see there, then the plane may fall, and crash, and burn. Lit by the moon, vast plains of snow and ice slide by below: we are approaching the Arctic Circle. Mountains of snow, pain, loneliness; sure death, slow and terrible. If you must look, see it as mere background decoration, stage design. This is how we do it—how it has always been done, in fact. During the winter of 1868, when the London workhouses were packed to their utmost limits with the destitute and the dying, the president of the Poor Law Board was on holiday in the South of France.

But what has that to do with us? We do not treat the helpless and the dying—rich or poor—in our own society in such a way. Or do we? Was there in fact a change in the way we regarded human beings, particularly the incurable members of the community, during the period we have been taught to admire as the Age of Enlightenment? And does this change still linger as an unacknowledged prejudice in the modern mind? One hundred years ago, my own grandfather's grandfather was growing roses in New England, reading Shakespeare to his children by candlelight: a gentle country doctor, a kind and courteous man. Did he know, I wonder, about the workhouses, the concentration camps for the unemployable and for the chronically ill, which in England—the land of his own cousins and his forefathers—had become the Dachaus and the Belsens of the day? Poor because they were sick, sick because they were poor, these were the ones who, if judged beyond cure, were turned out of the best London hospitals and sentenced to die in the workhouse. My grandfather's grandfather died in his own bed, at home. People did, in those days, if they could afford to.

But why the workhouse? Medical history suggests at least one answer. Doctors and hospitals were struggling day by day in England for the economic right to exist. And indeed, "what opinion would the public form of the skill of the medical attendants in the hospitals if upon looking at the annual reports it should appear that the cases of death were to those of recovery as three to one?"

Not a very good one, true. But doctors and hospitals were not having much success at curing people in those days; and in industrialized, Victorian England, disease was rampant, particularly among the poor. It was a dark time, a dark passage in medical history, the hygiene of Greece and Rome forgotten, the medieval knowledge of healing herbs and anodynes generally ignored. Polite people of the Victorian age took themselves very seriously and solemnly indeed; they spent a great deal of time congratulating themselves and one another (if they had solid bank accounts) on their respectability and their superior moral virtue. Propriety so smug has its daemonic side. Surgeons operated then not only without anaesthesia, but without washing their hands or their instruments. One London doctor, famous and much admired at the time, was proud to own a surgical coat so encrusted with blood and filth where he had wiped his scalpel over the years that when taken off, it would stand alone. A wiser physician named Semmelweiss, who insisted upon hygienic procedures, was driven mad by the mockery of his colleagues, and died in an asylum, disgraced. It was a great age of medical discovery and scientific experiment, but the comfort of the patient was no longer a main issue; and the Protestant work ethic had transformed incurable people into a scorned and unwanted class.

It was not only doctors who formed the public opinion of the day. There were few of them, and in their sometimes hideous fashion, they surely tried to serve society's interests as best they could. The question really was, what were the interests of society? Here, as usual, a clue can be found in the vocabulary of the day.

Individuals sentenced to workhouses were commonly referred to, in print and by respectable citizens, as *objects* or, on occasion, as *miserable objects.* The solid, well fed members of society died in comparative comfort at home while their fond families gathered around for the parting solemnities, waiting eagerly for the will to be read. Those who were mere objects, broken tools no longer able to serve the new mercantile system, were put away out of sight and, as much as possible, out of mind. Life in the workhouse was designed to punish the offender for the disagreeable crime of dying slowly, in a conspicuous state of disrepair, without funds.

How did this change come about? We know, for one thing, that Protestant clergymen since the Reformation had been preaching with great vigor the message that pain and sickness were a punishment for sin. The Puritans who migrated to America did not, unfortunately for England, manage to bring quite all of their savagery on this subject with them. Part of the transformation was religious; it represented a collapse of the medieval system of belief. Those who suffered were not seen now as holy, and no longer represented in their persons the suffering of Christ. Another reason for the change was economic and political, growing out of the circumstances of the Industrial Revolution. To be rich and dying in Victorian days was to languish in an entirely acceptable fashion; while to be poor and incurable was a sin. You could die of consumption or even of an unattractive social disease and, if you had money enough, expect deep sympathy, plus a marble monument over your tomb, draped with limp-wristed angels weeping; but if you were poor it was a different story. Disease in the rich was glamorous. In the poor, it was a sign of moral degeneracy.

We voyagers now being carried so lightly through space in a machine of the twentieth century, we who are so highly favored— what has all of this to do with us? Nothing, if we do not realize how precarious our position is, and how much of what we want out of life cannot be bought with money. How delicate is our balance, even at this moment—and the old man beside me coughs again, unconsciously, poring over the book he has brought with him—so that the simplest journey we make must weave its way always in and out of the real possibilities of instant darkness, present death. Each society chooses its own outcasts. Ours demands health and beauty, talent and power. Tonight we have it. But what about tomorrow?

And what about yesterday? Yesterday it was London, 1866. Snow on the ground, no heat, stone buildings pressing upon their inhabitants the cold of centuries, a pall of coal fumes in the air. Not in a plane but in a workhouse, people as real as we are lay crushed together then with stone walls on four sides and windows too high ever to open on any view. At Paddington (say the records of the day) one small towel was provided for 31 inmates—people with heart disease, syphilis, typhus, tuberculosis, and rickets, "the English disease." At Kensington 40 were forced to share 13 beds with iron strips across their frames—no mattresses. At Castlebar the diet was water pottage, with a sheep's head boiled occasionally for soup. At Maryborough ... At the Strand ... rats and lice, babies crawling half-naked on the cold stone floors, whimpering. But, stop! We are not strong enough to hear any more of this, even to think of it. How could such things have happened, in a solidly progressive "Age of Reason"? What, in this world, has become of *hospitality?* Where are the clean, soft linens, the coverlets and the cradles, the goblets of silver, the sweetmeats and the wine that were given so gladly in the old days to the dying: *the precious possession of the community, for heaven was open to them?* Where are the hospices of medieval times and where is *caritas?*

We are astonished and confused, because we have believed so thoroughly the myth that human society moves in a steady, upward thrust as time goes by, toward freedom and enlightenment. Our schoolbooks taught us that Victoria's England was full of petticoats and parasols, a little absurd perhaps in its solemn propriety, but at least reliable and solid in its basic values. And we were taught that people in medieval times were cruel, superstitious and quite barbaric; whereas we and our immediate ancestors, of course, have entered the Age of Enlightenment and of Technology, and thus have been able to accomplish such marvelous things as the Industrial Revolution, the rise of nationalism, the mercantile society, intercontinental missiles, napalm, DDT, and the Bomb. Hitler's regime, only 30 years after its downfall, seems already to us an anomaly, one of those odd little abberations that need not be explained, except perhaps as a footnote in some future textbook of history.

But it was during the Age of Reason that Napoleon melted down the goblets of the Hospitallers' patients to pay his armies for a megalomaniacal war of conquest. And in purportedly elegant nineteenth-century England, the cakes and the wine were in the mansions and private homes of people who quite honestly believed that they were better than others, purer of blood, more sensitive, deserving, and morally worthy, simply because they had more money. The reasons why they had more money were probably thought of as infrequently as they were mentioned; and to the proper Victorian, a great many facts of life were unmentionable. The theft of monastic properties by Henry VIII and his cohorts; "enclosure," which is to say, systematic, legalized robbery over the years of peasant agricultural lands; these of course were among the main reasons why there was now a huge class of vagrants and unemployed. Industry exploited these demoralized members of society who had once been yeoman, hardy, independent, and proud; it separated them not only from their land but from the parish communities of their birth, in its demands for labor pools at factory locations. Poverty seen from a distance can seem like mere background decoration.

Polite Victorians ignored conditions in the mine pits until they heard that women were working naked from the waist up, beside their men, in tunnels 18 inches high. Then they were horrified—by the suggestion of sexual indulgence that this scene implied. In the parlors of London, they knew better: they draped shawls over piano legs so that the sight of these naked appendages would not arouse their men to "beastly" behavior. Meantime, the factories and the mine pits of the day used men, women, and children less fortunate like machine parts, kept them unspeakably poor, and made them sick unto death. In this condition they were useless, and a blazing reproach to the moral consciousness of their "betters"; and thus, the dying poor became the American slavemaster's niggers and the Hitler's Jews of England, one hundred years ago.

The movie is over now. It was something cheerful, evidently, about pirates. The moon has moved below the horizon, or we, perhaps, have moved away from it; encapsulated now in our own night thoughts, we are surrounded by nothing but darkness. We know what time it is in San Francisco and what time it is in London, but here we have no way of measuring it, not knowing any more exactly where we are. Most people are sleeping, but not the elderly man beside me, who is so frail that his bony arm feels nearly weightless beside me, seems to take hardly any space at all inside his sleeve. He has large hands with long, thin fingers holding a worn, leatherbound volume of something—Homer, surely?—written in Greek. Slowly he turns the pages; each page, edged in gold, gleams briefly as it turns and settles lightly. His shoulders give a little shake and for a moment it seems that he is coughing again, but a quick glance tells me that he is only enjoying a small paroxysm of private amusement. Is it, I wonder, *The Iliad* or *The Odyssey* that he finds so refreshing? My own journey on this particular night, a breath away from him, must be a darker one. Tomorrow I will walk in at the door of St. Christopher's Hospice in London, and I am not sure yet how to find my way there. It is not simply a matter of locating a number 12 bus, or of hailing a taxi once we are on the ground again and giving an address. In order to be present at St. Christopher's, one cannot come from San Francisco via the Arctic Circle; it is necessary to come there from the medieval hôtel-Dieu via the workhouse.

History, I am thinking, does not work at all the way we were taught, does not rise in triumph like a rocket or a plane into space. It works more like an accordian, perhaps, expanding and then collapsing on itself; or like a loom with its shuttle riding back and forth, in and out of the threads already set: circumstance in a constant process of enmeshing itself with necessity. Most of its threads are thick and dull, but here and there are some with a curious brightness and a stubbornly shining quality about them.

These we must trace, if we are to perceive any pattern to the whole.

Reaching back once more, it is London, 1538. The monasteries have been shut down, their lands, their goods, and their means of hospitality parceled out, in the main part, among favorites of the king. The nursing orders are dispersed and no relief has been provided for the wayfarer or the needy sick, these past two years. People are dying in the streets and in the fields, untended. The citizens of London draw up a petition to Henry, entreating him to establish some place of refuge where the outcasts and the helpless may be "lodged, cherysshed and refreshed." These are shining words. They have life in them, the rustle of fresh linen, the smell of spice, the joy of bread and wine, and the warm promise of a human embrace. From these words we can tell that the citizens of London are asking, not for a house of correction, nor for a hospital in the modern sense, but for a place of hospitality—a *hospice*.

They ask, but from the state they do not receive. People who are irresponsible enough to be poor, it is thought, can be whipped into shape; and they are, by statute of Edward VI's coalition in 1550, whipped, beaten, chained, and branded for the crime of not owning the land that has been taken away from them and of being, therefore, unemployed. The weary stranger coming across the field in search of safety and shelter at sundown is no longer a *peregrino* or a *pilgrim*. The state has a new name for him now. He is a vagabond, and such persons, says the new law, "should be adjudged the slaves, for two years, *of any person who should inform against such an idler* ... and the master shall cause his slaves to work by beating, chaining, or otherwise in such work and labor how vile so ever it may be, as he should put unto him. . . ." The weighty self-righteousness of Victorian England, it seems, has begun in an outburst of fury, 300 years earlier, at those who do not fit into the new economic scheme of things. Better laws than this do appear later, and in time, a number of "voluntary hospitals" are founded to mend the bodies of the sick. However, for the time being a light has gone dim, and an essential grace has been lost. *Hospice* is no more. *Hospitals* during the seventeenth and eighteenth centuries express the desire of society for order, efficiency, and social discipline. As medical historian George Rosen says, it was "a humanitarianism of the successful, tempering sympathy with a firm belief in the sober and practical values of efficiency, simplicity and cheapness." Incurables were discharged from Westminster Hospital, founded in 1719 for the relief of the sick poor of that parish; and the governing board of Guy's Hospital took only eight years in finding a loophole in the will of Sir Thomas Guy that would allow them to do the same, although he obviously meant to offer shelter, in the name of Christian charity, to those very citizens. "Improving" tracts were left by the bedsides of the ill and they received, whether they liked it or not, a good deal of moral instruction, for the religious and spiritual care given in the early "voluntary hospitals" was "not that the dying body should give up a peaceful spirit, but that the recuperated body should possess a spirit less likely to fall a prey to idleness, drunkenness and other uneconomic abberations." The new unit of society was economic man. The purpose of hospitals in an industrial society is to mend machine tools, or to lock up separately those such as orphans, the insane, or the contagious, who may prove useful at some later date: hospitals as storage bins for society's spare parts. By the mid-1800s another purpose for hospitals is being mentioned. Approximately 11,000 patients in the better hospitals of London are now "beginning to be more carefully selected to meet the needs of teaching and research." Individuals fortunate enough to find a "sponsor" to recommend them for such purposes (and guarantee funeral expenses) are required to express public gratitude in the most humble of terms, for the exquisite generosity of their benefactors. The language of love itself is now corrupted. Sweet *caritas* has become cold and condescending *charity*, cautiously dispensed by the righteous to those who are clearly "deserving." *Dilectio*, drained of all joy, survives only as *diligence*—industriousness, imitation in one's daily, human life of a machine.

The golden thread is lost. How can we find our way? In fact we know that a way has been found, for attitudes toward the sick and especially toward the dying have changed radically of late; and hospices are springing up once more, in America and in the United Kingdom, specifically designed to give the best of medical and spiritual care to those members of society who are no longer useful to the industrial machine. And we can find traces throughout this dark age of a work that was being done, quietly and patiently, by hundreds upon thousands of individuals, in the simple name of love.

While seventeenth-century New England Puritans rejoiced in the spread of fatal diseases, which they had brought with them, among the Indians (the better that good Christians such as themselves should inherit the land), Protestants of a different temper went out into the streets of London offering goods and services to their suffering fellow citizens. Guilds already active in medieval days turned their wealth to the purpose of caring for their own sick and dying members. Conscientious individuals, such as Sir Thomas Guy, instituted a tradition of humanitarian philanthropy that crossed the waters later and became the basis for the American hospital system. Quakers risked and suffered persecution on both sides of the Atlantic in order to pursue their stubborn policy of treating all men and women, of whatever condition, as if they were indeed sisters and brothers. Augustinians, Benedictines, and other Roman Catholic orders continued their work on the continent, though often now under municipal or state supervision; and found their way back eventually into the fabric of English and of American life. Everywhere there were, as always, individuals who refused for private reasons to accept the popular moral attitudes of the day, and who continued quietly to care for their fellow human beings, making *dilectio* a noun of human action, and of loving choice. As hospitals have learned better how to cure people, many of these individuals have now turned their attention to the care of those who are beyond the power of science to mend, and whose time has come to make the final journey.

Of all the threads that illuminate the substance and the fabric of this time, one leads directly to St. Christopher's Hospice in London, 1976. Following its path we can move through four centuries of time, touching people who knew and touched one

another, and looked into one another's eyes, over the span of some
13 generations. First in this line was a French priest who was
captured by pirates and sold as a slave, shortly after the year
1600. After converting his third master to Christianity he
returned to France, and there founded a hospice for galley slaves,
an orphanage, a number of missions to the sick poor, and a
nursing order called *Filles de la Charité*. This man was Vincent de
Paul. His Sisters of Charity were taught that their monasteries
were the houses of the sick, and their cloisters the streets of the
city. For three generations, they went quietly and anonymously
about their work, bringing aid and solace to the rejected members
of society. Early in the eighteenth century one Baron von Stein of
Prussia visited the hospices they had established by this time
throughout France. The baron was deeply impressed. Back in his
own country, he wrote an eloquent public statement describing
the "expressions of inward peace, repose, self-denial and innocent
sprightliness of the Sisters, and their kind and benign treatment of
the sick who were entrusted to their care."

Baron von Stein's influence opened the way for a young
Protestant pastor named Fliedner to found Kaiserswerth, the first
Protestant hospital in history to have an order of nursing sisters,
or deaconesses. Kaiserswerth, like the hospices of the French
Sisters of Charity, was dedicated to the aid of the destitute sick
and the dying; and once again, three generations passed while the
influence of Kaiserswerth and similar organizations grew and
flourished on the Continent. In 1840 Elizabeth Fry, an English
Quaker, visited these hospices, including Kaiserswerth, and was
inspired to dedicate the rest of her life to prison and hospital
reform in England.

Florence Nightingale was a contemporary of Elizabeth Fry.
Rejecting the values of her proper Victorian family ("We are
ducks" they said, "who have hatched a wild swan"), she fled the
provincial and dilettante life they had planned for her, served
some weeks with the Sisters of Charity in Paris, and went on to
work for three months at Kaiserswerth. When she left for the
Crimea, Florence Nightingale brought with her nurses trained by
Elizabeth Fry, by Kaiserswerth, and by the Sisters of Charity; this

was a group drawn from sources both ecumenical and international: English, German, and French, Protestant, Anglican, and Roman Catholic.

We remember the thousands of wounded young lives she saved, and we see her still, the Lady with the Lamp, walking the wards at Scutari late at night, while soldiers blessed her and kissed her shadow on the wall as it passed. She brought cleanliness, fresh air, decent food, and passionate concern for the welfare of each patient as an individual, into a situation that had previously been a nightmare of filth and ignorance. She also established nursing as a profession worthy of respect, for the nurses of seventeenth- and eighteenth-century England had been, almost without exception, pitifully ignorant, incompetent, and in dire need of medical attention themselves.

However, Florence Nightingale's concern did not extend only to those members of society who were curable. She herself suffered during most of her long life from painful attacks of an illness which may have been psychosomatic, the product of nervous exhaustion in a body weakened at an early age by strain, and a personality which was far from the norm. "How little the sufferings of illness are understood," she wrote, "how little does anyone in good health imagine himself into the life of a sick person! ... 'What can't be cured must be endured' is the very worst and most dangerous maxim for a nurse that was ever made. Patience and resignation in her are but other words for carelessness or indifference." These are heartfelt words that might be taken as the motto of a modern hospice for today.

Florence Nightingale lived until 1910; and it was, in fact, one of the Sisters of Charity, her co-worker and contemporary, who founded in Dublin in the late nineteenth century a place of shelter for the incurably ill, and called it, in English, a *hospice*. Sister Mary Aikenhead was her name. Little is known about her, but she must have been a remarkable woman. The French still kept the name *hospice* for many of their shelters and orphanages; and it may have been that Mary had met this word during a period of training with the Filles de la Charité abroad. However, it is equally likely that, perceiving the dying patients she loved and honored as pilgrims departing on a longer journey, she chose for this reason to resurrect the gentle and half-forgotten, medieval English name.

Around the turn of the century a number of other hospices appeared in Great Britain—and in 1892, a "Hostel of God" in London which still exists—but the direct line now leads from Dublin to St. Joseph's Hospice, established by English Sisters of Charity in London in 1906. After previous training at the Protestant Hospice of St. Luke's (also in London) it was at St. Joseph's during the 1950s and 1960s that Dr. Cicely Saunders further developed her work in pain control and, together with some of the patients who had inspired and enlightened her during this period, her plans for the founding of St. Christopher's. In 1967, Dr. Saunders opened St. Christopher's Hospice, where I will be going to work today.

Women, it seems, have been a significant force in the hospice movement since its reemergence in the seventeenth century. Women, and a slave and a priest, a powerful nobleman, a poor country pastor, a Quaker, and a brilliant child of the upper middle classes who dared to rebel—what had all of these in common? All, for one reason or another, were outside the system. None of them found it alluring to think of themselves as mere objects—even as rich, socially prominent, and therefore very important objects, setting a solemn example of respectability to their inferiors. Many of them probably knew the joy of forgetting to think about themselves at all. Not having any investment in the mercantile and the material scheme of things, each was richly empowered to love God and do as he pleased.

And now I find that, while I have been tracing the golden thread, the plane has already begun its long, slow, and shuddering descent into Heathrow. Where has the night gone? Evidently I have been asleep at some time or another, although I don't remember it; but someone has done up my seat belt for me, and put a blanket over my knees. My white-haired companion has put his book away at last and is now apparently giving his entire attention to a buttered bun and a steaming cup of tea. Our journey is nearly over, and now it is too late for us to become acquainted. I feel some regret about that, wondering what his night thoughts have been like, and what book it was, actually, that he was reading.

The sky is very gray. Last night in London is already this morning—or rather, with nine hours missing, it is tomorrow afternoon. A cup of tea and a bun with jam somehow fail, as far as I am concerned, to fill the gap. The plane thuds and lurches down now, on the ground again, and lumbers along the runway to an unsteady halt, groaning and complaining all the way about its electrical deficiencies, its internal disconnections, its unfortunate set of tires, its leaky valves. We are gods no longer. Wet snow is falling from the sky, melting and vanishing as soon as it touches the ground.

Standing in line for Customs, I look out of the dim, stained window in the wall of concrete block, and catch a glimpse of our marvelous flying machine. By daylight in starry snowfall, it looks like a cosmic reject, something that happened a long time ago, in the days of the dinosaurs, perhaps, by mistake. And yet, what a sense of mastery, what a sense of power it has given us! A bird would laugh.

My elderly friend is standing beside me, and I am tempted to ask him whether or not birds laugh. He looks like the sort of man who would know the answer to that question. He stands with his hands thrust deep into the pockets of an old mackintosh, with a woolen muffler wrapped rather carelessly around his chin, and his lips pursed as if he might be about to whistle. Binoculars, I am certain, are somewhere in his luggage. He owns a small boat, I think, and putters around on it endlessly, splicing odds and ends of rope and making notes on the habits of sandpipers and terns. But he is not whistling, he is smiling. Our eyes meet directly for the first time, and I realize to my surprise that he is about to say something to me. His eyes, deep-set under coarse, white brows, are the curious color of sunlit amber, pale brown and flecked with gold.

He coughs gently, clears his throat and remarks, "You know, of course, what Chesterton said about flying?"

"Chesterton flying? Heavens, what a thought."

"Quite."

"But, what did he say? I would be much obliged—"

"It was in one of the later books, I believe. Flying. Yes. He said angels can do it very easily because—"

"Yes?"

"Because, you see, they take themselves so very lightly."

Delighted as a child discovering his first pun, he waits with beaming face to make sure I have got it—if I haven't, he will be more than happy to tell it again—and then, being an Englishman, turns with great delicacy away so as not to intrude upon my pleasure, and very soon, rather suddenly in fact afterward, disappears.

A Rare Combination

CHAPTER 6

Not only is [the hospice idea] novel to the high-technology big-business system of medical care we have, but it embodies a rather rare combination of spirituality and hard medicine, a combination whose uniqueness may not be appreciated until one encounters it in such a person as Cicely Saunders.

Constance Holden

I haven't worked in an institution before, and had heard stories of places where you couldn't just get on with the job but had to be careful not to do another man's work; here it is not like that. We are just part of the team and we don't keep arguing about whose job is whose, but we just get on with it.

Stan Phillips, Maintenance Dept.
St. Christopher's Hospice, 1976.

Surrounded by lawns and gardens in the residential district of Sydenham, some forty minutes by car south of central London and across the Thames, lies the cluster of brick and glass buildings known as St. Christopher's Hospice. Past a shared greenhouse space banked summer and winter with flowering plants, patients' rooms and wards in the central, four-story building look out upon trees and the rooftops of private houses nearby, and a busy neighborhood park with tennis courts. A play school for younger children of the staff (also frequented by older ones on holiday) is set just behind the main building and near a garden with footpaths, a reflecting pool and flower beds: a protected place of meeting in mild weather for children, patients, visitors, elderly residents of the "Drapers' Wing," and for the people of all ages and many nationalities who train, study, and serve in various capacities at St. Christopher's.

The outpatient clinic and the chapel are on the ground floor of the main building. Across the lawn beyond a neighboring private home is the Study Center with its library, its bookshop, its seminar rooms, and a small auditorium for films, lectures, and special demonstrations. Here also is a functional model of a St. Christopher's patient-care unit where students are able to learn techniques of hospice care by acting out the part of the one who is ill, as well as the part of the one who is offering assistance. Students live on the grounds together with many of the permanent staff members and their families, some in a residence hall behind the Study Center and others in a recently refurbished block of apartments nearby. To the arriving volunteer, it is a puzzle of major proportions at first to understand which is doctor, which is nurse, which is social worker, seminarian, psychiatrist, administrative assistant, steward, or secretary; and even in the wards themselves it is not always easy to be certain at first glance who is sick and who is well. St. Christopher's is first and foremost a community; and it is very much a village community of individuals.

At Sydenham Hill the air is cooler and fresher than at Heathrow in the west, or in downtown London. A light, dry snow has fallen here in the night and has clung, so that the main building of the hospice in its shell of glass is luminous throughout with reflected white. Large oil paintings, vigorous and glowing with brilliant color, are everywhere: the work of Polish artist Marian Bohusz, friend of St. Christopher's. Pine trees stand in the hallways today, decked with Christmas ornaments, many of which have been hand-made by patients and other members of the hospice community. Outdoors the sky is darkly gray at noon, seeming to absorb its only light from below. The roads and footpaths throughout the area are slick with ice. It is a good day to be inside, looking out.

Indoors, the stamping of snowy boots, laughter, the clink and clatter of kitchen pots, the fragrance of beef broth and rice, warm bread, Hungarian goulash. In the main dining room, lined with glass doors opening out into the garden, a few blue-uniformed nurses are already finishing their midday meal; one sits alone, staring in silence out at the snow. Men and women from the Drapers' Wing are gathering at a table near the inner door, some in wheelchairs, some walking together chatting amiably, others on the arms of visitors or pink-uniformed volunteers. These elderly people, frail and without families of their own to assist them, live in a group of sixteen bed-sitting apartments donated by an organization, active since medieval days, known as the Drapers' Company (Guild). If they become ill or unable to look after themselves with minimum help, full hospice care is made available to them on a temporary or a permanent basis.

The children troop in now, staggering and giggling, with their hands over their bright, scrubbed faces. Someone asked them what the joke is, but they aren't telling. Matron darts by in her gray uniform with its silver, heraldic belt buckle: Miss Helen Willans, who in America would be known as Superintendent of Nursing. Then Dr. Cicely Saunders, tall and smiling, moves from table to table throughout the room, stopping to talk briefly with a young woman who is evidently a doctor, then with an older man in tweeds (resident? relative of a patient?) and next, leans over the kitchen counter holding her plate and conferring at some length with a cook's assistant who evidently has something special on her mind.

The joke is out. It is George's hair. Whenever the young man, age five, takes off his cap in this weather, his fine, white-blond headstuff flies out in all directions and causes mild hysteria among the other members of his age group. Scowling, George pauses beside the wheelchair of a lady who is only a little larger than he is, although she must be well over ninety. She murmurs consolation and reaches out a bent, arthritic hand to try and smooth him. A young administrative assistant arrives on the scene and produces a dampened comb, which does the trick; and it turns out that the staff member is, in fact, George's mother. For several years now, working at St. Christopher's, she has been able to have lunch with her young son every day, and he in turn is in charge of running errands for her and keeping the thumb tacks and safety

pins sorted out in her desk drawer. This afternoon, residents of the
Drapers' Wing will sing carols and have a tea party with
members of the play school group while their parents continue to
work, under the same roof.

In volunteer's uniform now, I am sitting at a long table near the
garden with Dr. Saunders, Matron, and a mixed group of doctors,
nurses, and other volunteers. Conversation is quick and light, full
of cryptic little absurdities.

"Bird flew straight in at my window today."

"Left her card, I trust."

"Have you seen Sheila's new play?"

"Sat on my chair so I gave her a biscuit. Yes, marvelous. *Bed
Before Yesterday*, wasn't it?"

"Bed before what?"

"Tot of rum in her tea as well, I trust. Sheila Hancock, she's a
fabulous actress, and for you visitors, she's a member of our
Council here at the hospice, too."

"Britain and America are two rather similar countries—who
said it?—separated, unfortunately, by a common language."

"Mark Twain. Same chap said newspaper reports of his recent
demise were vastly exaggerated."

Laughing, we turn to the question of British and American
slang, trading stories about silly misunderstandings, and about the
bureaucratic jargon that so often serves, on both sides of the
Atlantic, as a substitute for thought; and now Dr. Saunders, like a
master chef tossing crêpes, turns a delicious phrase, catches it in
mid-air, turns it there into an even fresher bit of nonsense, and we
all explode in merriment.

The conversation continues apace, but Dr. Saunders is suddenly
quiet. She looks down at her plate for a moment in silence, puts
her napkin aside, and abruptly excuses herself from the table.
Returning a few moments later, she chats as agreeably as ever and
does not explain to me until later, in her office, what has
happened. "Mr. O'Hara has come in to us this morning," she says,
working absently at a large, red and black question mark on her
desk-pad, "after having been looked after by our Domiciliary
Care people at his home, until now." She reaches for another pen

and begins to outline the question mark in bright blue. "Mr. O'Hara is very poorly—very poorly indeed, and in fact, I am afraid that he will not last the night. As we were all having such a good time in the dining room, I realized that his wife, Mrs. O'Hara, was just coming in and I could not bear to have her think we were insensitive to her situation. I went to her and apologized."

"I am sorry. I am afraid I always laugh much too loud."

"But of course. So do I. Have done, all my life. It got me into a lot of trouble at school." She puts the blue pen down, then picks it up again and begins to draw symmetrical blue loops outside the question mark. "Mrs. O'Hara is a remarkable woman," she says. "She has had a great deal of hardship to bear, and she has managed it all with absolutely tremendous courage. They are a Roman Catholic family." She speaks now of each member of the O'Hara family in loving detail: a story of grief and struggle, triumph and loss. "She was very kind when I spoke to her; she would be, of course. She simply said, *"But I understand, life must go on. . . ."*

"The pictures you are looking at there are of David Tasma, the one who looks so young—he died in 1948—and of Antoni, who was Polish as well, and there is my beloved Mrs. G., and Louie, too. Patients of mine, all of them, my loves, my support system. Patients are the founders of St. Christopher's. It was through David's eyes that I was given the vision of this hospice, in the beginning. As he was dying in a busy surgical ward, we talked for many hours of what his real needs were—not simply for medical care as such, but for someone to care for him as person, to stand by and honor him for what he was—and it was he, a refugee from the Warsaw ghetto, who left the first £500 for St. Christopher's. 'I want what is in your mind and what is in your heart,' he told me. I saw then that what was needed was a place that was both a hospital and a home; and he said, 'I want to be a window in your home.' We have many windows here, as you see—look there, I think we will be having more snow, this afternoon."

"You had trained as a nurse during the war?" I ask.

"Yes, but was invalided out with one of those hopeless backs—it still gives me trouble, now and then—and I've had to spend quite a time lying flat. Gave me a great deal of time, of course, for thinking. I then did social science at Oxford, a war degree, terribly fast—ridiculous, really—but after David, I finally knew that I must begin all over again, and do medicine. That took some time. Eventually, I had a research fellowship at St. Mary's with a grant from the Sir Halley Stewart Trust to work at St. Joseph's Hospice with the sisters and the patients there, particularly in pain control, and to develop what I had already learned at St. Luke's as a volunteer RN from 1948 to 1955. Nurses have to work directly with the patients who are dying, you see, and they have always tended to be the leaders in this field. I saw at St. Luke's that you could take the doctor's prescription for medicine 'as required' and if you interpreted that to mean, 'as required for the control of pain' and not, 'when the patient is already screaming'— and gave drugs on a regular basis—then the patient's life was transformed.

"It was while I was training as a medical student that I came to know and to love Mrs. G. She spent the last seven years of her life in hospital, finally lost her sight, and was almost totally paralyzed but completely alert, full of joy and fun and interest in everything. She loved everyone about her and we spent hours together over the years. She died in 1961. That was a bad year. My father—I adored him, we fought madly—and Mrs. G. and Antoni all died, in one year. It was nearly too much for me. I got my bereavements so muddled up. But always at the worst, strength came—from God, through other people."

"I know that you are a Christian, and that St. Christopher's is very definitely a Christian foundation."

"Yes. We are not all Christians here, by any means, but our work is done in obedience to the Christian imperative. For me personally, it could not be done otherwise. At those times, in that bad year, when I would stop by the door of the ward where Antoni died, and think that it hurt too much, that I simply could not walk into that place again, I would look up at the Crucifix, and let it hold me. Then I was able to go on. I think there is a sense in which we help to complete the lives of those we love."

"Antoni?"

"Yes, above all, Antoni." She smiles in a way, with a radiance, that includes his living presence in the room. "I looked after him of course, but he said to me once, near the end, 'You must go now—I am looking after you, too.' It's part of the story that is not finished yet. When he died, Antoni smiled—and looked amused. I believe he was seeing some of the answers to the questions he had been asking throughout his life, meeting the God he had always believed in so strongly. And I am sure he knew, too, that in the work I am doing now, I would be comforted. Life goes on, as you see, at St. Christopher's. In death's very midst it goes on, and I think so very often it is brought into sharper focus here because of the presence of death. There are important ways in which we heal our patients, and in which they heal us. Healing a person does not always mean curing a disease. Sometimes healing means learning to care for others, finding new wholeness as a family—being reconciled. Or it can mean easing the pain of dying or allowing someone to die when the time comes. There is a difference between prolonging life and prolonging the act of dying until the patient lives a travesty of life. At St. Christopher's, we try to offer people space in which to be themselves. We hold fast, but with open hands; because sometimes the most important part of loving can be knowing how and when to let go.

"For nurses and staff it means leading a true life, because they are helping others, of course. Yet it means more than that, too, because people nearing the end of their lives have so much to teach others, about the nature of relationships and about the meaning of life. They drop their masks and do not worry any more about inconsequentials. Most of us rush through our days, never stopping to wonder at anything; and yet, every now and then, if we can back off from it as the dying do, and see life as a whole, we begin to understand that marvelous things are happening.

"We learn, for example, that time has no fixed meaning as such. An hour at the dentist seems like forever, but an hour with someone you love flies past. And yet, wait a little and look back on it. The hour of discomfort and anxiety is totally forgotten. What is remembered forever is the hour of love."

There is a knock at the door and a television producer is

ushered in. We are introduced, and it is explained that he is
preparing a documentary film on St. Christopher's. At the same
moment, the telephone rings and several staff members appear
with papers, messages, and questions. When Cicely Saunders
stands up in a small room, it is an event. It is not so much that she
is larger than life in the physical sense, for she is not really so
extraordinarily tall, and though obviously a member of the female
sex, she is slender where it counts. The power of her presence
depends partly upon its elements of contrast and surprise. Gray-
haired, keen-eyed, she wears today a dress of brilliant emerald
green and a gold chain necklace, and over it a doctor's white coat
with an ordinary nametag. As she muses on the past, recalling
memories of great poignancy, she communicates at the same time
a quiet and joyous confidence that is contagious; it seems for the
moment that she has all the time in the world and has never been
in a hurry. But when she is challenged by any present task, as
now, we see immediately the warrior spirit, the ability to cut
through nonsense and go straight to the point with tremendous
dash and verve. Here is a woman who has learned the skill (or
perhaps she was born with it?) of being resoundingly self-assertive
without sacrifice of delicacy or femininity. She will go to great
lengths to protect the sensitivities of others, but when her passion
for St. Christopher's is touched as it is when she deals with the
media, I can see a flame here that may burn, as well as warm the
hands. After twenty minutes of discussion, the producer is sagging
in his chair. "Well, if it isn't done right," she tells him firmly, with
a dazzling smile, "it won't be done at all." He nods, exhausted. It
will be done right.

The hallways are quiet, late in the afternoon, and the gray sky
has gone dark. I have hoped to meet Mrs. O'Hara, but have been
corralled instead by the kitchen crew—a fierce gang, fast-moving,
ruthless on the subject of absolute cleanliness, insisting that I must
get food to the patients *now*, darling, while it is steaming hot and
not next week, thank you very much. No, no, not there! Into the
pig bin with that lot, darling!
    "Pig bin?"

"Nothing goes back down to the main kitchen, touched or not, even a bottle of something that hasn't been opened. Never, never. Germs. Wouldn't be clean, you know."

"But I mean, is there an actual pig somewhere?"

"Oh, yes, we have a contract with a farmer. He comes and gets it. And when you are done there, darling, scrub the bottoms of the pans as well. Not that way. Here, use this. Has to be done right, you know."

I scrub the bottoms of the pans.

Faces in the ward. An elderly woman in a soft blue dress and shawl, sitting in an armchair with her hands clasped in her lap. Mrs. O'Hara? A young girl sitting up in bed in a pretty nightgown, rolling up her dark hair in curlers while she watches ballet on television. A huge man in a raincoat, plodding along the hallway—father or brother of one of the patients, perhaps? But he leans over, presses the button for the lift with his forehead, and then stands whistling as he waits for it, tapping his foot while his arms dangle limply from his sides.

No telephone bells, no buzzers, no loudspeakers here, calling doctors' names. No smell of antiseptic, though everything is spotless and the floor under our feet shines with concentric circles of buffing and polishing. No smell of fear or sickness, no glittering banks of steel machinery, no IVs, no flashing lights. No one is moaning or crying out in pain. Statistics have it that there is one staff nurse per patient here, but, looking onto the ward, it seems there must be more than that, because people both in and out of uniform are sitting, visiting and talking with patients, and no one seems to be pressed for time. The curtains around one cubicle are closed and I can see the feet of three nurses and doctors working simultaneously with one patient. A very thin old lady sits up in the armchair beside her bed while a white-coated woman doctor, stethoscope in pocket, leans an elbow on the bed, looking exhausted. They are chatting amiably and, after a few minutes, the doctor straightens up, gets to her feet, and helps the patient back under the covers. "This is the only place I know," Dr. Gillian Ford tells me later, "where patients continually ask you how *you* are feeling. I told her I felt rather poorly today, and she was very kind."

Azaleas, ferns, chrysanthemums, cyclamens, African violets. Two single rooms at the end of each hall, four beds in each large and airy bay, each with its own curtains that can be drawn shut, and each with its own furnishings around it—tables, chairs, armchairs, photographs, cards, books. Colored quilts, knitted coverlets, and plenty of down pillows on each bed. Fresh white linens, worn and soft. Letters, newspapers, cigarettes, lamps, baskets of fruit. A bottle of port and two glasses. A family of five walking by with a small, gray, and very nondescript dog padding agreeably along behind them on a leash. Beside the bed of an elderly woman in pink, a small girl is curled up in an armchair, sucking her thumb, and reading a comic book.

"Haven't you got it all yet?" the old lady asks, amused. The little girl takes her thumb out of her mouth and says cheerfully, without looking up, "Go away, Granny." Granny grins at me. "Some is born sweeter than others," she tells me. "That's what I always say. Some has to work on those thumbs years and years, getting the honey off." She cackles with delight. Her head is like a skull, dark eyes blazing out of it from deep in the bone.

"What's in the book, darling?" she asks.

"Nothing."

Granny cackles again. "What did I tell you? Nothing in the book at all, see? It's the honey she's after."

In the bed across the way from them is a woman—young? old? fortyish, perhaps?—lying very still. Her pale, blonde hair is streaked with silver, and her skin is so pale and fine that it looks translucent, glows in the light of the lamp above her like milk glass, almost like mother-of-pearl. When I speak softly to her, she turns her head a little toward me and smiles with great, blue violet eyes, welcoming my presence without question; says, yes, she is comfortable, thank you, feeling rather tired today, but she has been at home for several days and now she is resting, so that she will be strong enough to go home again for Christmas. She sighs a little, smiling, whispers something I can't quite hear, then sleeps, as I sit beside her holding her hand that is so frail and light that it is like holding a flower, or a leaf, or the memory of a human hand.

In the half light of the hallway beyond the next ward stands Dr. Thomas West, Deputy Medical Director of the hospice. Having read his articles about death and dying, and about St. Christopher's, in the English medical journals, I recognize him immediately and am not surprised to find that his voice and his presence express very directly the charm and the compassion of the inner man. He is giving his full attention at the moment to a woman who appears to be in great distress; he speaks very little and listens with care to her halting words. Yes, this is Mrs. O'Hara. Her husband is lying in the nearest bed, just inside the ward. He is deeply unconscious, emaciated, curled on his side like a child asleep. His skin is a dull, green gray, and he takes a slow breath once or twice per minute. Two grown sons and a young woman sit with a blue-uniformed nurse at the bedside, quietly watching over him.

"You did the right thing, Mrs. O'Hara," says Dr. West very gently. "He belongs here with us now, my dear, and you with him, and the rest of the family as well."

Mrs. O'Hara's face is grief. No armor, no defense. Tears well in her eyes as she speaks slowly, dazed, groping for words.

"He was better for such a long time. I am sure that he was. I stayed home from work and saw that he ate his meals. He gained some weight, too."

"You did a fine job of it, Mrs. O'Hara, a wonderful job. No one in the world could have done better."

Seeing my uniform, she turns to me and takes my hand as if to reassure me. "They came from here, you know—and helped us so much. At the other hospital they told me he had only three months to live, but when he came home he did ever so much better."

"Nine months it has been, hasn't it?" says Dr. West.

"Yes. And he liked to go out so much. Last week I took him to Dorset where he was born, and he saw the old house again, that he remembered. Only last week we had his birthday, and he did enjoy it so. He never had any pain, after the people came from here and he had his—you know, the blue medicine, and he started walking around again in the house. But yesterday morning it began again, and this time, it was so bad, I knew it was time."

"And then you called us for more help, which was exactly the right thing for you to do. You knew that we had a place promised here for you, whenever you should need it."

"Yes, and it was such weight to bear, heavy like lead, but I put it down at the door when we came. Now he is safe. The Father has been to see him twice, but oh, I never did get to Mass today, myself."

"Tomorrow then," says Dr. West quietly, putting his arm around her shoulders, and they walk together to the bedside. Mrs. O'Hara is an extraordinary woman and has managed well, but Dr. West's concern extends itself equally to those who prove far less able. "In fact," as he remarks later, "the more inadequate the family appear to be, the more marvelous it is, that they have coped at all."

For more than two years now, Mr. O'Hara has been ill with cancer of the stomach which has spread, despite radical surgery and a course of chemotherapy, throughout his intestinal system. At home, visited by the Domiciliary Team and by district nurses advised by St. Christopher's medical staff, he has been active and comfortable with the help of a round-the-clock, four-hourly prescription of the "blue medicine" (in his case, most recently this has consisted of Diamorphine Hcl 20 mg, Cocaine 10 mg, Stemetil Syrup, 5 ml, and Chloroform Water 10 ml, plus prednisolone 2.5 mg 2 tid to help him maintain his appetite). After a massive hemorrhage he has lapsed gradually into unconsciousness, and death is now imminent. Since his arrival at the hospice he has been gently bathed, dressed in a clean gown, and made comfortable; no medication has been given except his regular narcotic by injection and intramuscular hyoscine 0.4 mg to dry up the excessive secretions which tend to accumulate when a patient is dying. Thus, there will be no interludes of choking to disturb him, and no "death rattle" to distress those who are now watching and waiting with him.

The curtains around Mr. O'Hara's bed are not drawn; life in the ward continues and the nurses go by on quiet feet, but do not avert their faces. Dr. Saunders has been making her way through the wards visiting with patients and checking on details of their medical care for several hours now; she stops for a quiet moment with Mrs. O'Hara at the bedside here, says something to the nurse, and touches the arm of each of the O'Hara sons lightly and affectionately, before moving on. Most of the other patients in this ward are now sleeping, including one elderly soul who evidently prefers, for some stubborn and private reason, to sleep sitting up in an armchair with a quilt over his knees. Time passes. Beyond the black windowpane, flakes of snow like feathers float, lift in the wind, and seem to spin out from the light, into space. Every now and then, Mrs. O'Hara leans forward and strokes her husband's forehead, smoothing his hair back as he breathes. The time between his breaths is very long now, as if he were a man so preoccupied with the measure of his own stillness that the occasional breathing in of air has become an unwelcome interruption, a punctuation mark unnecessary in the flow of his private contemplation.

Time. I lean my forehead against the cool window, and my breath mists the glass. Again, I do not know what time it is. A car passes, silent in the snow, its lights searching. When I look back, I see the nurse taking Mr. O'Hara's pulse, and then Mrs. O'Hara suddenly reaching for the nurse, gathering her in a silent embrace. Heads close together, the two women sit for a long moment. Mr. O'Hara looks the same. The only difference is that he is not bothering now to breathe any more.

The nurse kneels down at the bedside and they all kneel beside her. This is the moment when simple, traditional prayers are customarily used for each patient at St. Christopher's, for says Dr. Saunders, "few families do not want to accept the offer of this commendation." Mrs. O'Hara holds her dead husband's hand in both of hers and rests her head against it, as they pray. It is not like sleep, I think. It is something else. Pilgrim, fare well.

"That's the way I want to go," says Mr. Pippin to me in the morning. "Nice and peaceful. Not that I'm ready yet, mind you, for I've seen them come and go, and I am still here enjoying myself, which suits me fine. Do me up, will you, love? Yes, he had a fair and easy riding of it, he did."

Mr. Pippin is the tall, round man who whistles in the hallway, "Believe Me If All Those Endearing Young Charms," like the true Irishman he is, on his mother's side. He cannot use his arms, so I fasten up his fly for him while he tells me about the musical comedy he is going to this afternoon in London. A volunteer will come and fetch him in her car. "Drives like blazes, she does," he says with anticipatory glee. "She'll have me there in less than thirty minutes."

Mr. Pippin is riddled with cancer throughout his spine; however, he tends to ignore the patient's role and has become instead inspector general, ombudsman, and purveyor of cheer to all in the community. If a patient needs a spit pan in a great hurry after breakfast, it is Mr. Pippin who tells the new volunteer exactly where to find one; he then takes it upon himself to make certain that the patient does not sit around feeling sorry for himself after having chucked up his morning toast and tea. When two nurses bicker over the morning change of linens, Mr. Pippin appears on the spot to tell them they are both looking prettier than ever today and he doesn't know how he will choose between them. "Mr. Pippin," asks Dr. Saunders, "what would you say to Matron that she should look for, when she hires a nurse for us? What is it that a nurse should have, first and foremost?" "Patience," he replies instantly. But there is a gleam in his eye and I wonder if I have heard him right. No use asking Mr. Pippin however; he would only give us a wink and be off, down the hallway again whistling "Believe Me If All Those" and flourishing his grand red beard that came, so he says, from his mother's uncles before him. Hauls himself along now like a seal on a rock, Mr. Pippin does, yet in spirit is light as a hummingbird, sipping a bit of fun here and there, poking his head into everyone's business, teasing, enjoying, tasting the mischief, the marvelous fragrance of life, and everywhere, pollenizing.

Day by day his ponderous body becomes more helpless and more useless to him, and therefore receives less of his notice. He

likes it all right—admires his beard in the looking glass with a sort
of absentminded, familial affection—and yet, the heavier his limbs
become, the more Mr. Pippin himself is lighter, will not be bound
down or pay homage to danger, embarrassment (only does up his
trousers at all now, as the Duchess said, so as not to frighten the
horses) and one day the news will be, without doubt, that he has
achieved transformation into something finer and more delicate
than ever, having slipped, with a grin and a wink at this world,
from his cocoon.

The news in the nurses' lounge at all hours is fatigue. Also, the
price of food in London (terrible), the difficulty of giving up
smoking (worse), and the patient's husband (unspeakable) who
prevents their twin daughters, age seven, from seeing their
mother now that she is dying of cancer. The social worker has
tried, the psychiatrist has tried, Dr. Saunders herself, it is
rumored, has tried to help the man deal with his situation more
sensibly, but he will not. He does not want his daughters to see
"ugliness" and he firmly believes that they will "forget" the
anguish of having their mother leave them for no understandable
reason. The nurses are irate. They chip and peck away at the
image of this villain who somehow grows larger and more
menacing each time he is mentioned; and in their talk there
appears to be a venting of general frustration, and of the anguish
of caring so much as these women obviously do, for patients who
die. Is it exhausting work? I ask.

Of course it is draining, they reply. And yet, surprisingly, it is a
tremendously satisfying job as well. We natter on about it because
that's just the way we are. But we know we are relieving pain
which is simply not coped with in other places where we've
worked. We see them coming in to us in terrible shape, in agony,
many of them, and some of them with bedsores neglected and
other infections. We clean all that up. We get them comfortable,
free of pain, get them to eating, feeding themselves again (many
have been on IVs), and see them sit up in their beds, get up, and
move around again when no one thought they ever would. Most
of all, we see them part of their family again. Some go home and

then come once a week to the Thursday clinic. Most of them can at least go out again on visits; and that part of it of course is marvelous. We are well paid here, too, salaries the same as National Health standard for work that is in many ways not as hard, because we have more time to do it in.

The frustrating part comes when sometimes there is a run of such terribly ill ones coming in all at once, and then dying before we have a chance to do very much for them. There was a time like that recently in fact, a "bad patch" in the summertime when it was unbearably hot. When they come in and die straightaway—as with Mr. O'Hara—it is mostly for the family what we do then, being with them so it is not such a frightening thing at the last. And we'll stay in touch with Mrs. O'Hara of course, and the rest of the family, if they'll come to the Monday evening meetings we have. But the hardest thing of all is, getting very much attached to one or another of the patients, particularly the young ones like that Mrs. Preston who was just confirmed and had her first communion here only last week.

We meet once a week with some of the other staff and once a month, you know, with Dr. Colin Murray Parkes (psychiatrist and author of a number of works on bereavement). Between them and ourselves we get things sorted out. Some of us go to the chapel and have a cry. And we do fume and fuss somewhat among ourselves as well, getting it out—taking it out, some might say. But the doctors know how we feel, and Matron, and they feel it too. We're all in it together and we are a team, that's the main thing.

"You wouldn't prefer to work somewhere else, then?"

"Not after what I've seen here, I wouldn't."

A network of meetings blueprints the inner workings of St. Christopher's. Staff meetings, ward meetings, doctors' rounds which in this case are more meetings; meetings of residents, council meetings, meetings of the bereaved, and meetings that cross the lines back and forth between various groups which, in other institutions, might coexist without intercommunication. There is even a Thursday meeting with a bar set up for patients and staff (including maintenance men) especially to share. After morning prayers for those who wish to participate, one of the most important meetings of the day is held regularly in the Admissions Office. Here, hospice principles are put daily to a test of definition and redefinition that is a constant, and at times anguishing, reminder of the delicacy and the difficulty of St. Christopher's chosen task.

In the small room crammed with desks, filing cabinets, and records, six people must sit almost knee to knee in the space remaining, while they struggle over the applications that have been submitted to the Hospice. Matron is here, the Admissions Secretary, her assistant, the chief social worker, and a member of the Domiciliary Team. One by one, each individual is discussed on the basis of the report submitted by the attending physician, a report taking into account not only the medical situation, but geographical location, family relationships, life style, present state of mind, and any personal problems which may have developed during the course of illness. Nearly all have cancer.

How are they chosen? Of six who may apply in a day, it appears that only half may be tentatively accepted. It matters, first of all, that there is pain—not temporary, not easy to manage, but chronic and overwhelming to the individual. Other symptoms persisting despite previous medical treatment are also studied with care. Second, the individual should have some reasonable hope of life expectancy beyond hours or days, and should have relations or friends within reach of transport to St. Christopher's. The question is often asked, can the Domiciliary Care people manage to take on the care of this one? However, this is a difficult question in itself, for home care brings with it the assumption of a bed at the hospice when needed, and this cannot *always* be so.

Mr. Jones, it seems, would probably do better at home just now. The real issue here seems to be that his daughter is anxious to return to her position at the bank, and does not know what to do with him in the meantime. St. Christopher's cannot address itself to this problem, but will participate, if wished, by advising. The Admissions Secretary agrees to talk it over at greater length today, with Mr. Jones's social worker.

More information is needed on a number of cases, before any
decision or recommendation can be made. Referrals to other
hospices or nursing homes are given in several cases of people at a
distance, and arrangements are made for consultation with the
attending physician if wished. The case of Mrs. Smith now arrives
at the top of the pile. Already in a hospital under the care of a
GP, Mrs. Smith has suffered many months of devastating pain,
dyspnea, and other complications of incurable cancer of the lung.
She is deeply depressed and, when conscious, hysterical. Her
prognosis: days, or perhaps hours. Her doctor, contacting St.
Christopher's for the first time today, hopes for an immediate
telephone call, and a transfer on the spot.

Members of the committee look at one another aghast. The
social worker squirms in her chair, twisting her long hair between
her fingers, the Domiciliary Team member sits white-faced and
grim, biting her lips, and Matron, bolt upright as ever in her
immaculate uniform with its gleaming silver buckle, looks ready
to spit bullets. The agony of Mrs. Smith hovers in the room like a
vulture. "We cannot do it," says Matron. "No, we cannot." There
are 54 beds in the hospice. Every one is now either occupied or
promised to someone whose problem, in days and weeks past, has
intentionally become St. Christopher's own. St. Christopher's is a
house of life and of conscious, orderly transition for pilgrims on
the longer journey; its integrity as a hospice depends upon its
stability as a community. The time of transition requires medical
and nursing expertise, love, intelligence, faith, cooperation, hard
work. The physician in this case will be telephoned immediately
and given information which, it is hoped, may be of service to
him as well as to his patients, present and future.

The remaining applications are discussed. In each case, there
will be a response offering some kind of consultation, aid, or
advice, for each individual involved is a matter of concern for this
group. At last, Matron jumps up from her chair saying, "*Yes.* Yes,
this one sounds right for us. Indeed, I do think we can help her."
She beams like a small girl who has just found the finest Easter
egg of all. "You see, this one—Mrs. Green—she needs to be at
home for Christmas, but then will be ready to come to us for a bit.

Her family are quite close by, good transport, several more months, they expect, needs help with her appetite, partial paralysis, anxious and troubled, pain now increasing—oh yes, we can help her. A sound, conscientious report from her GP and he understands what we are about at St. Christopher's. *Good. Mrs. Green."*

Money is not mentioned during this part of the Hospice proceedings. St. Christopher's was established in 1967 as a charitable foundation, and although at present some three-quarters of daily, patient-care service receives support from the National Health Service, other costs and working capital must come entirely from gifts. Public appeals for funds are not made, and it is through families and friends of the hospice that the majority of its financial obligations are met. There have been desolate moments when the budget (now nearly £600,000 annually) has seemed impossible to meet. Thus far, some donation or renegotiation of funds has always intervened; and no patient has been turned away from the doors of St. Christopher's for lack of money.

Had money been an issue, the woman who shall be called here Lillian Preston would have been turned away. Names, personal histories, and identifying characteristics of all patients here are, of course, thoroughly disguised. They speak, however, in their own words as I heard them, and as I believe they wanted to be heard.

Lillian Preston, age 29. She was the only child of aging parents, reclusive and impoverished gentlefolk. Married at 22. At 23, abandoned by her husband. Unable to find work, left with a baby daughter to care for, she returned in disgrace to the grudging parental home. Job finally found as a decorator's assistant in London, a two-year struggle ensuing, to establish a home for herself and her daughter. Success at last; and then, on their first holiday together, a boating accident in which the child is drowned. Six months later, Lillian Preston's doctor tells her that she has cancer, and that her uterus must be removed. Her uterus is removed, and after surgery, she is told that her cancer has metastasized beyond hope of cure.

Mrs. Preston looks now like a woman in her late forties. She sits
in a pale yellow quilted dressing gown, writing notes, in the
armchair beside her bed, her abdomen swollen as if she were
eight months pregnant. She has long, dark hair, bones like a
racehorse, dark eyes and eyebrows, very white skin drawn taut
over her cheekbones, an aura about her that is not quite a trick of
the light—a radiance. Prognosis: two weeks.

We talk of this and that. I clear her tray, help her into bed.
Tomorrow the doctors are going to draw off some of the fluid, she
tells me, and then she expects to be more comfortable. Now?
Well, not too bad, really, only she is so heavy with it, and rather
sleepy. Strange to feel so peaceful, so secure now and almost to
feel—well, happy, really, even though she knows—she tests my
eyes—that she is not going to get well. It is such a relief, she says,
not having to pretend any more. It was so hard, more than she
could bear for a very long time, being alone with the knowledge
of it.

"Had you no one to turn to?"

"No one. After I was ill I had to stay with my parents again,
you see, and my father wouldn't hear of it."

"But, your mother?"

"He insisted on protecting her, you see."

"So you knew that he knew, and still—?"

"No one would let me talk about it. It was a horrible secret that
everyone knew and no one would mention. And the worst of it
was being so helpless, a burden on everyone. It was like having to
be a child again, only worse, because they would say, soon you
will be getting stronger—and this time, I could not. So I let them
down, again and again, and I could see them actually hating me
for it despite themselves. Then I started hating myself. Until I
came here, I used to hope each night that I wouldn't wake up to
live another day. Each hour seemed like a week, each day was
like months. And when I was in the other hospital, I had to have
morphine shots to knock me out for the pain, but that isn't living.
When it is that way, you really can't call it being alive. The
psychiatrist at the other hospital was very kind and he tried to
help me, but he couldn't give me what I needed."

"Then it is very different here, for you?"

"Here I am treated as a person. I have a sense of my—dignity. Well, I don't mean that, it sounds so proud, but here I am simply myself, and no one minds. I am glad to live each day now, one at a time. I like to nap in the afternoons, but I am so busy here, it is actually hard for me to fit that in. So many people—friends I didn't know cared for me, people I used to work with—have written to me, come to visit me and so forth, now that I am here and it is all right to say what is happening."

"How long have you been here?"

"Nine, ten weeks I think. Perhaps longer, I don't remember. It's strange, I hardly even remember the pain. I remember the fact that it was so bad, I could not bear it. . . . Yes, it was physical pain, and also the sense of being such a failure, having lost out on everything I tried to do. And the grief of losing the one child, the only thing that mattered. The pain was terrible, but I think it was grief that always made it past bearing. I was angry too. At the world and at life, and most of all, at myself. And then I came here—have you seen how it is when we come? When we arrive? Matron comes straight into the ambulance, the moment it stops in front of the door. She does that for everyone. And she came in to me, and called me by name. I looked at her face and could see that she was glad to have me. It seemed as if she had been waiting, only for me. That is why I am always so near to tears here, it is such a relief. And all that time, I never believed in God. Can you imagine? Listen, a week ago something happened that was very strange. I felt in the night the Angel of Death, it seemed. In my sleep. It was the presence of death just by my shoulder and I thought, this is my time to go. But it was not. It was the woman in the bed just there beside me, she, who died that night. But I felt it, and I went up out of my body and floated above it. I knew I was in my spiritual body then, and I was not afraid, but I was glad to come back because I am still not ready. I have to work through things in my own mind that are not finished yet. Here at the Hospice, you see, things are so different from all that I am used to. I have to go over my whole life again, it seems, sorting it out. Do you think that is strange?

"You don't," she continues. "Well, that is one reason why it is so good to be here, where no one thinks I have gone mad. Let me show you something—I hope you don't mind this—but I want to show you what it was like before." She pulls back the sleeves of her nightgown and holds her arms up to the light. The scars I have seen, but never like this. Most people, when they cut their wrists, only want to bleed a little and frighten the people around them into being kinder. Lillian Preston has savaged herself, wanting to die.

"I did that," she says, shaking her head in wonder, putting her arms back under the coverlet again. "It never did heal right."

"When was it?"

"Before I came here. They sent me to one hospital, then to another. Then, when I finally came to St. Christopher's, the young man—you know, the chaplain's assistant—he came to me and we talked about it all. He helped me."

She closes her eyes and lies very still, smiling slightly, pregnant with her own death, pondering her memories, biding her time.

Now There's Tomorrow

CHAPTER 7

You matter because you are you. You matter to the last
moment of your life, and we will do all we can not only to
help you die peacefully, but also to live until you die.

Cicely Saunders

Sunday morning: a faint ray of sunlight gleaming in the chapel.
On the long wall, a spare and simple cross, two branches of cherry
wood from a nearby tree. The altar is not, as might be expected,
at the far end of the room but at the side and center, so that we
can bring the beds into a semicircle around it; and those who are
too weak today to sit upright can still see and participate.

Packed as the chapel is now with beds, wheelchairs, patients,
residents, visitors, and members of the staff, the scene is distinctly
medieval. Once more we are able to experience at firsthand the
time in history when the ward of a hospice-hospital was in itself a
holy place. In the monastic way stations of the twelfth to
sixteenth centuries, the ward with patients lying in it was shaped
like the nave of a church, and was in fact just that, arcaded beside
the patients' beds and opening directly to the vaulted apse
beyond. The cross-shaped plans of later hospitals were not
originally designed for ventilation or for the convenience of the
medical attendant; their original purpose was to allow as many
patients as possible to witness the Mass and to participate in
communal prayer and worship even while desperately ill or

dying. The fact that the cross shape proved also to be useful in a practical way is one of those events, like Mr. Pippin's puns, perhaps designed to make us think.

By comparison with the fifteenth-century ward of the Hospitaller Knights at Rhodes which had its altar at the side, presumably for the same reason, this room is small, modest, and austere. And compared to the lovely and gracious old monastic wards at Canterbury and Tonnerre, even at Turmanin in Syria in the fifth century A.D., it is indeed very plain. Yet the same life goes on here, now as then. And in its obedience to the Christian imperative, to heal, and to come together for healing, it is a commanding room in the very power of its intimacy.

We sing a hymn; or rather, Cicely Saunders sings a hymn, and the rest of us do the best we can with it. Actually the sound of us all giving it a try together is not bad. People in bathrobes are singing, and people dressed, and people lying down in nightgowns and pajamas singing, *a cappella*. The human voice, even in such a situation as this, is a fine and hopeful thing. For indeed, it is strange, as Mrs. Preston might say—her favorite word, "strange"— to see people lying down dying, singing. But why is it strange? What is it that we have become used to, instead? There she is now in her yellow dressing gown, lying back against her pillows, dying, singing.

Strange means alien, unrelated, foreign. Foreign to what? Strange means being a stranger, being away from home, coming across the fields at twilight, weary, needy—or coming across the Arctic Circle in a plane, frightened, in the night. Strange means needing to know what time it is, and not knowing. Not being able to find your way home. Where is home? To the stranger, the dogs at his heels in an unknown town are strange. He knows who he is, but they do not. Let them hurt him enough in the hour of his anxiety, and he may become a stranger to himself, unrelated, alienated—mad. But who in the world we live in today is mad? Is it madness to live with the sight of, and in the knowledge of, death and dying—or is it sanity?

I want what is in your mind and what is in your heart, said

David Tasma. He wanted both a hospital and a home, bread, not a stone. What is home? Bread and wine and singing. Home is where the music is. Hospitality, like music, opens out a space where we can come together whole, heart and mind, and love, and be healed. And in this space there is not any here, nor there, nor boundary, nor judgment, nor distance set between us, nor any way of measuring who is a stranger; and in this space, because there is no measuring it any more, there is no time.

World without end, amen. The brief Anglican service, built around the moment of Holy Communion, is concluded, made miniature so as not to tax the strength of those who are very frail; for Sunday at the hospice is a day of many visitors, excitement in the wards, children and pets, cousins and grandparents in the hallways, gifts and flowers arriving, and general celebration. The lifts are busy now, taking beds back to their usual places, the front door of the hospice is opening constantly, and the telephone at the reception desk is jingling.

The honored visitor in Dr. Saunders' office today is a cheerful and expansive lady by the name of Dame Albertine Winner, who is Chairman of the Council of Management at St. Christopher's. A physician herself as well, and formerly Dr. Saunders' Deputy Medical Director here, she obviously cares very deeply about each challenge and problem within the hospice, though she claims it is all mere pleasure and holiday, pure delight for her, coming on weekly visits to talk with anyone available, seeing an occasional patient in consultation—her particular joy—and working with other members of the Council. These she finds fascinating in themselves; representatives of the church, the theatre, the law, business, banking, medicine, and social work as well as individuals with a special dedication to voluntary service. Matron attends these meetings also, as does the bursar of St. Christopher's and the architect; thus there are knowledgeable and experienced leaders in many fields, from the larger community as well as the hospice itself, available to inform and advise one another in all matters relating to the development of St. Christopher's. Dame Albertine's connection with the hospice began in 1961 when, as

Deputy Chief Medical Officer in the Ministry of Health, she first
saw what was being done for patients at St. Joseph's Hospice. At
that time, she became a firm supporter of Dr. Saunders' plan for a
place which would not only look after patients' needs, but be a
center for teaching and research as well, and an ongoing
community. A founding member of St. Christopher's Hospice, she
has been its resourceful and determined advocate ever since.

It was 16 years ago, when these early conversations between
Dr. Saunders and Dame (then Dr.) Albertine Winner took place.
And it is now nearly 29 years since the first vision of St.
Christopher's was given through the eyes of the dying young
refugee from Poland. The young doctors gathering together with
Dame Albertine, Cicely Saunders, and Dr. Tom West today must
have been, some of them, in their cradles then. Yet between them
all, men and women, younger and older, there is an easy
camaraderie and a sense of great mutual affection. In time for
ritual libation before Sunday lunch, a bottle of sherry appears,
and a set of stemmed glasses from the cabinet surrounded by
books. Cicely Saunders pours. "Who will carve at Christmas this
year, Dr. Saunders, in the wards?" asks one of the younger
physicians. "Dame Albertine will, and Tom will of course, and
now that you mention it, you will too," she replies with a grin.
"Cheers."

"Do you never rest?" I ask her. We are driving toward London
in the four o'clock afternoon darkness and I am acutely conscious
of the fact that in San Francisco, this morning for most people has
not yet begun. It is raining a little now, as we approach the
Thames.

"Oh yes," she replies. "I was so exhausted yesterday that I went
home and slept eight hours straight. And I am on my way to a
party now, with some of my Polish friends. Hospice work is very
taxing, as you see. I believe it should not be embarked on at all,
unless one is the sort of person who really cannot help it.
Someone, preferably a doctor, must be prepared to be a leader,
have an overpowering desire to get it going and be prepared to
sweat and pray to do it. But we in this work, I think, are always

somehow missing one layer of outer skin, and we must take care to renew ourselves. It must be done from within, by means of prayer above all, but celebration as well. The work of a hospice must be done right, and its spiritual dimension cannot be grafted on. We must have ideas in order before it is possible to meet facts. Yes, I do rest, and I celebrate, and I thoroughly enjoy myself in my small private life which is tucked away, around the corner from St. Christopher's."

She drives steadily, competently ("I find it restful to drive") at a fine clip straight down the wrong side of the road, which turns out, of course, to be the right side after all. The right side of the road, in the world we now inhabit, *is* the left side. *Looking glass world,* as the American doctor visiting said today, speaking of hospice care and comparing it to the treatment of the dying cancer patient in hospitals of his own country. And his question was, how is the decision made, when to move through to the other side, where automatic attempts are no longer made to conquer the disease, but instead, every effort is brought to bear in support of the person's physical comfort and spiritual well-being?

The reply was that these are in effect two complementary systems of treatment, and that there should be openness and interchange constantly between them. The attending physician, in consultation with the patient and the family, must take it upon himself to make the decisions—and may, if there is doubt, call in consultants—but must always be on the alert to prevent the patient from becoming locked in to a system which is inappropriate to his needs.

"A patient should no more undergo aggressive treatment, which not only offers no hope of being effective but which may isolate him from all true contact with those around him, than he should merely receive control of symptoms when the underlying cause is still treatable or has once again become so," said Dr. Saunders. Patients suffer not only from inappropriate active tumor "cure" but also from inept terminal care, of course. The aim of a hospice must be to rescue the individual from both of these destructive alternatives. "The work of a hospice is to give

patients the attention they need; it is a job equally demanding as
that of a more conventional hospital but involving different skills,
more personal. But it's good, hard medicine all the same."

Personal, yes, I think the following morning, kneeling on the
bathroom floor, powdering between the toes, one by one, of Miss
Aurelia Robbins. Skills very personal and involving the most
minute attention to detail at the same time that the mind is being
stretched to its utmost limits in the opposite direction, toward
infinity. Only in the life of the individual patient, the body and
soul of each person, seen one at a time very clearly, and with
great care, can these opposites meet. Hospice care, like life itself,
is not a thing but a process. Terminal care is not really the right
word for it, does not suggest at all the right kind of tension, the
balance here between left-brain, right-brain matters. Miss Aurelia
Robbins's left foot is rather different from her right foot, and yet,
she needs both of them, to walk.

Walking, she sees herself, still (and likes to tell me about it) in a
garden in Charleston, South Carolina, in the spring. There are
lilies of the valley and hidden violets under the trees, and she is a
young girl, with her hair up for the first time, wearing a white
dress. It is 1920, and the people in Charleston are very, very kind
to her. She does not know how she could ever thank people,
really, for being so kind. The air is warm and soft in Charleston in
the spring, and she walks under the trees in her white dress, every
day, never forgetting to tell me how kind these people are,
because she knows that I am an American too. It is a great
pleasure to dry Miss Robbins' feet, and to put powder on them.

"You have beautiful feet, Miss Robbins."

"Do I really, my dear? Why how nice to think of that, because
you know, of course, I haven't seen them in years." Miss Robbins
is blind, and the skin of her face is crumpled like an old rose, but
the skin of her body which she has not seen for so long is like a
young woman's, innocent and smooth, wholly unconscious of
itself. She sits in the deep, warm tub and says, "Ahhh . . ." when I
squeeze the sponge over the lovely, blind skin of her back, and
smiles a marvelous smile. Miss Robbins has been at St. Christo-

pher's for seven years now, first as a resident in the Drapers' Wing and then, being unable to care for herself any further, she moved into the wards of the Hospice. "I never married," she says. "Wasn't that selfish of me?" She likes her lemon cologne after her bath, but she needs to be reminded that she likes it. Looking inside her mind is like looking into one of those glass baubles that you shake a little, and the snowflakes swarm, and then they settle down again, and grow still.

Sitting up today in her chair in her soft, peach-colored dress and her little shawl, with her hands clasped in her lap, she smiles and says, "I'm just an old fraud, you know. I'm not even sick at all. I am just sitting here enjoying myself. Isn't that terrible?" Then she tells me again about the kind people in Charleston. "I don't quite understand it, really," she says. "Life is a great puzzle to me, but I think there must be a meaning to it all somehow, don't you?" Miss Robbins does not know it, but she is a challenge to the word *meaning*, as a rose is. She wants her cup of tea if it is there, and if it is not there, then she does not want it. Anything that might have happened to her in her life, and did not happen, was superfluous. She very simply enjoys being. Mornings, she says, "Oh, how nice of you to suggest a bath. I do love being bathed and I always forget, but you know, people here are so kind, they always remind me." Then we go into the bathroom again and I squeeze the sponge over her back, and she says, "Ahh . . ." and tells me again about Charleston. Americans, she says, must be really the kindest people in all the world. She does not wonder whether the people in Charleston have forgotten about her, or whether, in fact, they may be already dead. She does not want any more from them than they have already given her. She takes her pleasure now in offering her memory of them back as a gift, again and again, to me—the American—so that I, a stranger and far from home, will feel valued and cherished. Thus I, the care-giver am cared for daily by Miss Robbins, am bathed and cleansed of my strangeness, my foreignness, and am welcomed, made at home. Thus she, who is unable to help herself, heals me.

Miss Robbins is not known as "the senile glaucoma in 45-B" when hospice doctors meet for rounds. She is known, with great affection and appreciation, as a special person who has made for many years an important contribution to the stability of the community. Her condition will be carefully watched from day to day by skilled physicians and well-trained nurses, but it is the person and not the physical or mental disability which is of concern. Is she able to live her own life in her own way at the moment? Does she enjoy her meals? Is her radio working? Is there anything more we could possibly do for her? But then—and they smile—what could anyone do for Miss Robbins? Except, of course, to enjoy her, as they do.

This weekly meeting is held, not at the bedside, but privately, in an office. X-rays are discussed, chemotherapy, radiation treatment, and a certain kind of crutches that might be more useful to Mr. Jackson than the ones he has now. All patients, unless they specifically request to have it otherwise, are known by their family names with the appropriate title; in England, more than in America, this is felt as a mark of consideration and respect. Changes of medication are noted and discussed. Mrs. White has shown signs of discomfort and has been vomiting, thus she is now being given her analgesic by injection. Mr. Strauss has complained of cramps in his legs. Does he need hot packs, a different kind of orthopedic support, passive exercise perhaps, some subtle shift in medication, or a combination of these? Has he been successful in finishing his project in occupational therapy? Does his family celebrate Hanukkah, and if so, has he been fully involved in the celebrations? Knowledge is pooled, and it is decided that Dr. West, who is particularly close to Mr. Strauss, will have a talk with him about the changes that are planned in his regime.

Mr. Pippin's latest X-rays are "a disaster." He has had radiation treatments in other parts of his body, and has appeared to be holding his own. Suddenly now, his upper spine is in great danger, and it is a serious question whether he should go to his dear old friends at Shepherd's Bush for Christmas. A great day has been planned for him and all his godchildren; he has been looking forward to it for months, and it would be another sort of disaster if he were not allowed to go. This may be Mr. Pippin's last Christmas. But what would it do to the family and to the godchildren especially, if their merry, whistling, red-bearded god of a godfather should suddenly collapse in agony, or even die on that day in their midst? Could the family manage? Would they feel forever after that they had been somehow to blame? Would the children have a horror of Christmas in the future, if such a thing should happen?

After a lengthy discussion a decision is made, to provide a particularly sturdy and extensive neckbrace for Mr. Pippin immediately; then to have him transferred on the day itself by ambulance, only for the celebration, and then to return. "Oh, Mr. Pippin," says Dr. West to himself, looking sadly at the X-rays. "Look at that, the entire structure disintegrating! Yes, my friend, you are an amazing man."

"What are you doing, writing a book?" A patient I have not seen before has noticed me, standing beside the flower sink, scribbling notes. I help her back from the lavatory and into her bed and say, yes.

"About the hospice, I suppose. Why, how absolutely splendid, my dear. It's amazing how little people know about this sort of thing. Do you have them in America? Not that there's anything in all the world like St. Christopher's. Be an absolute angel and hand me my wig while you're at it. Cicely Saunders is a very dear friend of mine. Fabulous woman. Sit down this minute and let me help you write your book. . . . Oh, the wig is in that little box up there. Right, that one.

"Thank you. Not that I give a damn what I look like, but I'm going to a concert downstairs. Don't want to frighten people. Chemotherapy, you know. I've had cancer for ages, lots of secondaries and all that sort of thing. A frightful bore, really."

She is a large woman, Mrs. Kent, with the manner of a casual duchess rambling through her kitchen garden, philosophizing about aphids. She has a falcon's eyes, however, and probably rushes around Scotland—or used to—during the season, doing things with shotguns and stirrup cups. At home she undoubtedly has a closet full of floppy hats and floppy wigs, more or less indistinguishable from one another. Heavy silver on her table, and a great many large dogs under it, crunching bones during formal dinner parties.

"Have I got it on straight? Well, never mind. About this book of yours. Splendid. Everyone should be told. Hospices should be everywhere. All this talk about euthanasia is absolute nonsense. Well-meaning, of course, and I do sympathize, but the fact is, you don't have to kill people in order to make them comfortable. Look at me, for example. Not that I am anything unusual, though I am somewhat lopsided here and there, having bits and pieces chopped off of me hither and yon, but who cares about that? I am alive and enjoying myself. Every single person in the world should have a place like St. Christopher's to go to, when things get out of hand. I was absolutely howling with pain when I came in here, 48 hours ago. Hadn't been able to hold food down for nearly two weeks. This morning, I ate like a horse. Feel quite fine, at the moment, and plan to go home again in about three days. All I needed was getting my medicines adjusted, and having a bit of rest. Tell them that. Personal experience, my dear, believe me, the only kind.

"They know what they are doing here, you see. They do miracles, I assure you, but not as a result of floating about in a sort of euphoric trance praying and all that sort of thing—not that I mind if they do, at this point—but it's all a result of absolutely tremendous discipline. And the moment you come in here you feel you are the only pebble on the beach. That in itself is the most incredible lift. Write your book and tell them everything about it, for I am perfectly certain as I sit here, that hospices are the coming thing. . . . How did I happen to know Cicely? Well, just as you do. I was once a volunteer."

Off in a wheelchair she goes now ("Don't need it, really, I'm just constitutionally lazy.") to the concert of Renaissance carols in the Draper's Wing; and I learn from Matron that an emergency situation has developed. An unexpected patient is arriving, a woman who has been until recently in a London welfare home that has been shut down. It had been hoped that Mrs. Doe could manage at home until after Christmas (in a filthy flat which she fiercely refused to leave) but she has "had some trouble" in the meantime "needing to be sorted out." There is no space for her, but somehow space will have to be found. "We must put Mrs. Doe into a temporary situation, which is not at all the preferred way of doing it," says Matron cheerfully, "but it can't be helped. She is our patient, and she needs to come in."

The ambulance arrives, and backs up to the glass doors. The doors are opened wide. Mrs. Doe's bed is already waiting for her, just inside, with her name on it, with fresh white sheets and coverlet turned back, and four down pillows. Two hot-water bottles in knitted covers have been warming the inside of the bed for Mrs. Doe and are still there, where her shoulders and upper thighs will rest. Crisp and smiling, Matron hurries out—this is her moment of joy—climbs into the back of the ambulance and bends eagerly over the cot. From the cot comes the sound of a small animal wailing, and I see her put out her hands to stroke it.

The drivers are tall and powerfully built, one male, one female, in similar uniforms, blue gray, with caps. Very fast and smoothly now, some 20 feet from the back of the ambulance to the warmed bed, they bring the cot. The object lying on it, which does not appear to be a person, is wrapped in a red blanket. The drivers flex their arms, rub their hands, and then very fast but very tenderly, begin the lift from cot to bed. The thing in the blanket screams. "There, there, dear," Matron whispers, bending close. "Everything is going to be all right."

Together we turn the blanket back. The smell is of unwashed flesh, sour incontinence, rags, vomit, and beer. Inside the blanket is a loose, gray mass of flesh and bone with matted hair. Objects such as this are seen sometimes at night, in alleyways of cities, propped beside the garbage cans. Hurrying feet of frightened and respectable citizens step past them, and in the darker shadows nearby, there are rats. It is hard to tell, really, whether these creatures are dead or alive. One hopes—but then, in such a situation, what is there to do?

Matron strokes the matted hair and says, "Mrs. Doe? Do you

know where you are? You are at St. Christopher's Hospice now, and we are going to take care of you." We slide the blanket out, and pull up the top sheet and the coverlet. Another scream, and a babble of words, incomprehensible.

"Well, goodbye now, Mrs. Doe," says one of the drivers. "Don't you worry any more, sweetheart. No one is going to hurt you here." Calling to the drivers that they must stop for tea or coffee if they wish, Matron whisks the new patient's bed away; I help her slide it into the lift; the door closes, and they vanish upstairs.

Back in the kitchen again, scrubbing the pans, I see Matron darting past an hour later, in the hall.

"Oh, my," she says, merry as a cricket. "They have put you to it, haven't they?"

"Oh, Matron, how is Mrs. Doe?"

"Settling in very nicely, thank you. Such a dear lady. She will be fine."

"But I thought—is she desperately ill?"

"Desperately ill? No, she is not." Matron is moving so fast that I must nearly run, alongside.

"She isn't? But I thought she looked—well, as you say here, rather poorly."

"Poorly, yes. Circumstances have not been favorable."

"I was concerned. Will she be better tomorrow?"

"We shall see." She stops so suddenly that I nearly collide with her. "Mrs. Preston wants her tea now, I think. It would be very nice indeed, if you would take it to her."

"Why how nice of you to suggest that, Matron. Mrs. Preston is a particular favorite of mine, you know."

"I know that," she says, glancing up at me with lips held perfectly firm and straight, but with the merriest eyes.

"It's the strangest thing," says Lillian Preston, lying back on her pillows in her yellow gown, sipping her tea. "I mean, how different it all is here, from what I am used to. I have so much to learn and have learned so much already, even in a little time. Today was a bad day for me, you know. I talked to Matron about it. They drew the fluid off yesterday and I thought that would give me strength somehow, but it did not. I am thinner but I am weaker even so. It made me cross. So I have been in a 'bad patch,' being tired of all these things my body does to disappoint me, feeling low and down, and taking it out on everyone around me. I was mean—well, I hope not mean, but really disagreeable today at least six times before breakfast, and then when I saw the same old mashed-up food I have to eat now, I was cross to the person who brought it to me. The chaplain says it is wrong to brood about the things you have done wrong, it is only a form of pride, thinking that you ought to have done better, not really a way of loving God and being sorry. He says don't dwell on it, just tell Him that you are sorry, and try again. But when I think of it that way, then I know how proud I really am, and then I brood about that.

"Being confirmed, I suppose, was the dangerous thing. I mean as far as the devil is concerned, that is really the last straw. Oh yes, I believe in the devil and I ought to know, for he has given me a very bad time. Being confirmed put him into a real fury about me, and now I am being tested, you see. The temptation for me, I am sure now, has been to believe that I would be perfect from now on, and that all the people around me, being so kind as they are, would be perfect saints. They are only human beings, though. And they will do things that make me cross, and things that I do not like. They even make mistakes, sometimes. Love is the thing I have been learning. Love that accepts people the way they are. I have to do it now and it is a terrific struggle. But you know, I think it is the reason why I am still here. It is something I have to know about, or else my whole life has been wasted. And the only way I can really know it is to do it myself, no matter how weak my body is, just care for people and love them the way that they are. I never knew that kind of love before. I never had it given to me, so I never knew what it was like. Loving the baby, seeing her love me, was the closest I came to it. But we never really had a home.

"So now I try. And I go back over everything in my mind, and I think, sometimes, why couldn't people's homes be more like this? A hospice shouldn't only be a place you come to when you are very, very sick, do you think? I had a dream the other night. It was so strange. I dreamed about a place where I was not sick, I was well, and still I cared for people exactly in this way, and so did they for me. After that dream, I thought perhaps it was a kind of vision, perhaps that is what it is like on the other side of things. Thy Kingdom Come. I love sleeping now, I dream of dancing and swimming and all the things I am not strong enough to do any more, all the things that I love. Do you dream in color? I never used to, but I do now. I never used to remember much of what I dreamed. I suppose I will be there soon, and then I will really know. More and more of me is on the other side now already. I am getting out of balance with it, and it is harder and harder to come back now, so uncomfortable here, with my body. Another week, perhaps. I will make up my mind, when I am ready. See how proud I am still? I am really very stubborn and proud. It is lucky I know God loves me in spite of that, isn't it? Oh, I am getting tired now."

I put away her tea things and help her to lie down comfortably. Leaning against the side of her bed, holding her hand, I am resting too. She holds my hand, and I hold hers. With her eyes closed, she says, "When I get there, I will ask them to make things ready for you."

In the morning, my last day at St. Christopher's, she is still sleeping. I scribble a note, and leave it beside her bed, glad that she is sleeping, and that we do not have to go through the ridiculous business of saying goodbye. Mr. Pippin is sporting a carnation in his buttonhole and a vast neckbrace that has caused some hasty renegotiation of his beard. Holding court in an armchair, he entertains a young, pretty volunteer. Miss Robbins has her bath, and tells me about Charleston. I powder very carefully between her toes. In the hairdressing room there is a new face under the dryer, small and pink, with very bright, blue eyes. Mrs. Doe is nowhere to be seen, but Mrs. White has stopped vomiting and is being a grouch, while the chaplain sits patiently beside her, nodding his head from time to time and sipping a cup of tea. Granny is having a nap, but I cannot find the pale, blond woman with skin so fragile, with skin like mother-of-pearl. Perhaps she has gone home for Christmas already, or perhaps—?

"Why hello there, darling," says a cheery voice, as I wander by with a watering can, tending the plants.

"Good morning, how are you?" It is Blue-eyes, from under the hairdryer, silky white sausage curls not yet combed out, peering from behind the morning newspaper.

"Sit down here for a minute, I'll tell you," she says in the rich accents of East London, a village far from the purlieus of Oxford or Cambridge, Harvard or Yale. Shaking her newspaper, she says, "I'll tell you it's shocking, it is!"

"Shocking?"

"Murder and robbing, that's all they do nowadays. Look here! What's the world coming to, that's what I'd like to know. Where're you from dear? America? California, that's part of Detroit, I know that, I've a nephew out there. You're a long way from home, then. Oh, well, times is hard now, dear, for all of us. I've seen some trouble myself, I can tell you. I've been so poorly, you wouldn't believe. I was bad with the pain, as God knows, though not being religious."

Her face is round and pink, and very clean. She wears a look slightly puzzled, inquiring, but pleased; and a fresh, flowered nightgown with a touch of lace at the cuffs. Every now and then she pulls her upper lip down and touches it delicately with her forefinger, adjusting her teeth. "As God knows," she says, "it's only a matter of speaking, for you'll never see me in a church. Day to day's how I live, do the best that I can, but so poorly, these six months my legs wouldn't hold me and now, here they tell me, tomorrow I'll get up and stand on my own feet again. How is that? This is some kind of place. You work here? Yes you will, wait and see, they says, that's what we're here for, to help you. Well I never. Why do they bother with me, that's what I'd like to know? Now, you answer me that. Look at me, nothing left. Lost three stone, have a growth down in there, ready to do me in. Nothing for it. Do me in, doctor, I says, I see your white coat, I'm ready. You'll feel different tomorrow, he says, and him holding my hand. Oh, well, now there's tomorrow.

"So, what for, I says, I am nothing but trouble. And where does it hurt then, they says. Well, it don't hurt any more today but I'm tired of it, look at me, ready to quit. Why are they caring, I'm asking? Why are they kind? I've got nothing to give them. Sooner's better to end it and not be a bother to others, if anyone stopped to be asking me. Which they didn't. No, not them. Some kind of a place this is, I'll tell you. They know I am done for so why give the likes of me—look, dear, you see my new hairdo? How is it? And get up tomorrow? Well, maybe I will, then, who knows. Maybe I'll fool every one of them, said I was nobody. They know my name here, look at that, put it right up on the bed. Had it waiting for me, when I was that poorly. But get up? I'm asking myself, how is that going to be, on these legs? Who would say such a thing as that? See here what I mean? These legs are no good. Well, come on now, just look at me, darling."

"Yes, Mrs. Doe."

This Passionate Concern

CHAPTER 8

The classical deathbed scene, with its loving partings and
solemn last words, is practically a thing of the past; in its
stead is a sedated, comatose, betubed object, manipulated
and subconscious, if not subhuman.

J. F. Fletcher

"General," murmured the tactful clergyman at Ulysses S.
Grant's bedside, "your time has come and the angels are
waiting for you." "Waiting are they," roared the General,
"waiting are they? Well, Goddamn 'em, let 'em wait."

Apocryphal

The elegant professor at the suburban dinner party is astonished.
"I simply cannot understand all this fuss and bother about
hospices," he says. "This incredibly painstaking method of care—
though I understand it is far less expensive than keeping vegetable
personages alive on drips and tubes—but why this passionate
concern with the care of the dying when it is so patently obvious
that longevity and surplus population are the real problems
confronting us? Do you realize that in 1900 only 4.1 percent of
the population in America was over 65 and it is now something
like 10 percent and rapidly climbing? We are going to be a nation
of arthritics and drooling dodderers by the year 2001. And look at
the energy crisis. *Your* energies, if I may say so, are being sadly
misplaced. Look at India. What the world needs is far more

people dying every day no matter how they go about it. Not to
mention, far fewer of them being born in the first place. Look
here, if we are to survive at all . . . and, we wouldn't be in the
catastrophic mess we are in today if only . . ." Thus he continues
with great verve and eloquence for 15 minutes or so to expound
the theory that all this hospice talk is incredibly sentimental; and
that another Noah's flood would be the best thing possible for the
welfare of mankind and (no chauvinist, he), with a bow to the
prettiest of the ladies present, of womankind, as well.

Professor N. is a sly man, sparkling with the sort of apocalyptic
wit that makes people gasp a little before they burst into
appreciative laughter. It is a pleasure to watch him as he
expounds and expands, embroidering and elaborating the more he
is applauded, enjoying his own eloquence, his own vigor as much
as he enjoys the handsome company and the excellent Cabernet
Sauvignon of his host. Waiting to hear (since we are suffering
from a rather serious drought in California at the moment) what
more practical solutions he may have for the population problem,
I note, however, that the space around us somehow shrinks while
he talks, and the darkness beyond looms larger, filled with
shadows now and with shapes becoming stranger and more
menacing by the moment. The world he conjures up is crammed
to the brim with people not like us, people out there called
"them" and called "they." These are individuals whom we do not
know and will never meet face to face, it seems, if we can avoid
it; but never mind, when the waters rise—we draw closer together
in our little circle of candlelight—when the flood does come, we
and people like us will be all right. Professor N., without quite
saying it, implies in his charismatic way that it will only be the
others, the nameless, faceless ones, who will die, while we here
with him now, so bright and full of *joie de vivre,* rejoicing as we
are in wine and quiche and candlelight, will survive; and that he
will be our leader in the wilderness, his wit our Ark. The magic
moment lingers on, for who could be so crass at a time like this
and in such blessed company to suggest, even in an apologetic
whisper, that our dear Professor N. does not know what he is
talking about?

He does not, of course. He believes that he is talking about the population problem. "Look at India," he says, waving his arm vaguely toward the shadows in the corner of the room. But looking at India does not solve the population problem; and in any case, Professor N. is not looking at India. He is looking at the people across the table from him. He wants to know whether we like what he has been saying. I for one have a hard time concentrating on what he is saying, however, because I am trying instead to listen to him. When I listen to him, I hear sòmething just under the surface interrupting the conscious message in a steady whine; I hear that he himself is now approaching the age of 65, and that he is bitter about his own life, and that there are a great many people in the world he is afraid of. I would like to ask him not to be so afraid, for I don't think serious, long-range plans are best made out of fear. Yet it is going to be very difficult to approach him in this respect. The people he is afraid of are all "out there" and there are a great many of them, all quite mysterious and invisible: invisible, just as Professor N. is at the moment, to himself. He can look down, I suppose, and see his hands, one wearing a thin, gold wedding ring and the other holding a glass of good, red wine. But in order to find himself, charming, witty, and important as he really is, he must look again and again, searching, into our eyes.

Am I amusing? he asks us silently. Am I wise? Are you glad that I am alive? *Am* I alive? Am I worth it? We gather close and, laughing, enjoying him, say, Yes, the guest is worth his salt. Reassured, he himself laughs, embraces us with his eyes, and continues with his plan for the improvement of humanity which is really his system for persònal avoidance—chivalrously including us, of course—of death. It is death who is his enemy, the death which he sees as personal obliteration, having dressed it in the foreign shapes called "them" and "they." But he does not know these people; and therefore does not know what he is talking about because he does not know *who* he is talking about. I wonder whether Professor N. might have happened to see a *Pogo* comic strip a few years ago in which one of the characters reports from the front lines in some bewilderment, "We have met the enemy and they are us."

I make a firm resolution (knowing that it will crumble) to

refrain from launching a counterattack in defense of the hospice concept. People who become deeply involved in hospice work, I know, tend to wear a kind of glow about them which at its best represents a healthy release of positive energy, but which can flare up all too easily into something resembling fanaticism. This is counterproductive, even though it is not difficult to see why it sometimes happens. Participation in this work is apt to produce exhiliration because of the changes we experience in our perception of such crucial matters as love and time, sickness and health, birth and death, and journeying, and the meaning of life itself. In receiving the dying as significant and fully conscious members of the hospice community we are at the same time reincorporating the awareness of death into our own lives, and this is a liberating form of illumination.

A hospice does not address itself to many problems of politics and economics which are indeed very pressing today—but then, realistically, neither does Professor N. What the hospice does offer, I am thinking, is a sane position from which to approach these other problems, since it is a position soaked through with reality; and at the same time is an affirmation of the value of human life which does not permit shadows in the wings, or self-deceptions about the comparative importance of "us" and "them" and "they." We are all going to die; death is in fact the great democratic leveler. The hospice acts out and embodies the provocative assumption that we are all one family responsible to one another in the meantime. Thus, though it does not preach politics, it is in itself a political as well as a philosophical statement.

"All philosophy," our host remarks, "is a preparation for death. Montaigne, wasn't it?"

"He stole it from Plato," said the professor. "Selective plagiarism, the *modus operandi* of the classical tradition."

"The *modus* of evolution as well," remarks the scientist, "if you want to have a look at the behavior of genes and chromosomes."

And (I am wondering) isn't it true as well, that the awareness of death—one's own death—is the best possible preparation for living? Knowing that we are going to die, we refuse to fritter away our time on nonsense, we drop our masks, our little vanities and false ambitions and, like General Grant—to hell with politeness—we say exactly what we mean. General Grant was madly in love with his cross-eyed wife, and I always liked him for that. He didn't necessarily disbelieve in angels, he just didn't want anyone standing around his deathbed being smarmy about them. He was busy dying his own death, and didn't take kindly to being interrupted. To live fully, as warriors know, is to embrace life in all its transformations; and here, of course, is the hospice idea again. In its power to incorporate all forms of human life—young, old, healthy, sick, witty and dull, feeble and vigorous—into one working organism in which each part is useful and nourishing to the other, the fully-realized hospice community such as St. Christopher's is a paradigm of what a more highly conscious human life might be, and of what society might therefore become. This was the vision of the young woman who was called, in an earlier chapter, Lillian Preston—she is dead now—who learned only in the last weeks of her life, in a hospice community, to love and be loved. And yet she is not obliterated, in the sense that Professor N. imagines that he will be. "The communication of the dead," said T. S. Eliot, "is tongued with fire beyond the language of the living."

Remembering Lillian Preston, I decide that I must try at least to say something. With her letter in my pocket, written to me only a few hours before she died, the spoken word will come hard. And only this morning the other letter came to me from the chaplain's assistant: "She died very peacefully, quickly, on the Sunday and after the Blessing when she herself had determined that it would happen. She was herself to the last, and never faltered in her faith, or in her caring for everyone around her."

To hell with politeness. If sentimentality, I finally manage to say, is "unearned emotion," then sentimental the day-to-day care of the dying is not. Furthermore, anyone who imagines that he is being terribly kind and noble in doing it is almost certainly doing a rotten job. The dying give us so much more than we could ever possibly give to them. And part of the misunderstanding here is that many people think of a hospice as being only a rather specialized medical facility or a fancy nursing home, but it is not. How would I define it? Well, I have a letter in my pocket that says it ever so much better than I could do. My friend at St. Christopher's says, it is a *caring community.*

Religious? Well, yes, if you believe that a caring community is necessarily religious. But in one very fine little English hospice I know of, two nursing sisters quit recently because they felt not enough religious ritual was being observed; and the director (who is both a physician and a deacon) asked them in astonishment, "But aren't you in the habit of praying with your fingertips?" So you see, it all depends really upon your own point of view.

Why are they necessary? Well, I suppose that a hospice is an expression of the fundamental urge to cherish what we value, and as far as I know, every culture worth the name has been built on the premise of valuing human life. Even the Neanderthals buried their dead with ceremony, and with flowers. But it is something else, too. It is also the embodiment of a recognition, deeply felt in almost every age and every culture since the Neanderthal, that life is a journey which will be continued in some other fashion, after death.

The word itself? Yes, I do think it is important. *Hospice, hospital, hostel* and *Hôtel-Dieu* were at one time such similar concepts that the words were used quite interchangeably, and only became separated later. This is the sort of separation, in fact, that has worked continually to fragment our society. The word *hospice* means a great deal to me because it is closest of all in our language to the ancient root: *hospes,* the mutual caring of people for one another.

With the growth of medical understanding, people who have contagious diseases have been separated more often from those merely in need of food and shelter, and this makes sense. However, the person who was dying, whether of wounds or disease or in the natural course of events (which we now see as unnatural!) was perceived throughout the medieval period as a pilgrim, a traveler at a way station on the longer journey. As early as the twelfth century the hospital-chapel form, developed within the monasteries, began to be imitated beyond cloister walls. But here too the dying were honored, and were tended with great care, whether their hosts were friars or nuns, or guilds, or princely benefactors. Inns sprang up as a commerical venture meantime; but for many centuries, kings and princes rubbed elbows in the courtyards of monastic hospices with the humblest of their subjects, and knew them by name; these were places of meeting for all sorts and conditions of people, and places of true *hospitality.*

If there has been a Dark Age (and if Professor N. will bear with me another moment) during the past two thousand years in the history of hospitality, in fact it has been ours. It was not until the religious and political upheavals of the seventeenth and eight-eenth centuries that such a different view was officially taken of "incurables" and that such an institution as the workhouse for the dying poor could appear. The treatment of our own dying, both rich and poor, in too many general hospitals today seems to me to derive from a curious amalgam of this new, mechanistic, and materialistic view of humanity, together with our neurotic, modern inability to face the facts of death. Our treatment of those who can be cured has grown a great deal better in the twentieth century; but the way we cope with our terminally ill has grown at the same time ever so much worse.

"You are a Don Quixote," says Professor N. "You tilt at progress, and at technology."

"Not at all. No, only at the ways in which we have misused it. Having invented machines, we had no good reason to begin imitating them, to let them control our thoughts. And having known better for thousands of years, we had no business suddenly deciding that the true model of a man's life is the machine which 'lives'—which is to say, *works*—and then, when it runs out of energy or is broken beyond repair, 'dies.' We know now that it is energy that is real, and matter that is mere.appearance. But the modern hospital deals with human life in terms of the material and the mechanical model. The modern hospice reaches back into the past and recovers our lost heritage; but its thrust is toward the future."

"You make a serious mistake if you do not respect the

mechanical model," replies the Professor. "You bury your head in the superstitions of the Middle Ages and forget the stink of the Hôtel-Dieu in Paris, which kept its doors open to every stray and every disease, and ended by piling people six and seven to a bed. The filth of that place was one of the scandals exposed by the military during the French Revolution."

"It was filthy, you are right. But *you* make a mistake if you do not recognize the fact that industrialized nations, once they get any power at all, tend very quickly to solve their own problems of population control, so that your vision of Noah's flood is, if I may say so, rather more primeval than medieval. I didn't hear your recommendation of what to do with all the bodies after the water goes down. There was a delightful letter once, in some newspaper or other during the Vietnam War, in which the writer suggested that it is quite all right to kill people in a civilized society as long as you plan to eat them afterwards. No, I do not at all condemn technology, and it is clear that it can help us in many ways. In fact the modern hospice can do a great deal better for its patients, on account of science and technology, than anyone could do at the Hôtel-Dieu in Paris in the eighteenth century. But let me choose another example in all fairness, because it was the condition of the sick and the poor at that time which after all caused the Revolution to begin with. The nurses who worked themselves to death there were trying to deal with a situation which was already, for reasons beyond their control, completely out of hand. But compare St. Christopher's today with, for example, the really exquisite Hôtel-Dieu in the city of Beaune, a hospice built in the fifteenth century, generously endowed with income-producing lands by its patrons, designed by the finest architects of the day. Its long chapel-ward for the incurably ill and the dying is one of the loveliest rooms ever to be constructed; its courtyards, its tapestries, its galleries—"

"Oh, you are a dreamer! Who pays for all this?"

"Who's paying now?" says his wife. "You are paying, I am paying, we are all paying, not only doctors' bills but insurance this and insurance that and lab fees, and tests that are absolutely useless because the doctors are all afraid that somebody is going to sue them for malpractice if they don't do them, and now we are paying for all those malpractice suits with more insurance, and higher fees, and when we get through all that we have to pay for everybody else when we pay our taxes. If I have to pay anyway, believe me, I'd rather go to some place I like, when my time comes."

"Pass the brandy," says Professor N. "Please. Where is Beaune? That's in the South, isn't it?"

"We never go anywhere," says Mrs. N. "I want to go to India."

"You would not like India, my dear. You imagine that India consists of the Taj Mahal by moonlight and a great many shops for you to buy beads and necklaces in. Like my adversary here, you romanticize; but if you were actually to walk the streets of Calcutta and smell the medieval odors there, you would be appalled, and I would have to prevent you physically from adopting two dozen grimy orphans who—"

"And I would do it, too."

"I know you would. And you would bring them back to San Jose, California, and set up a hospice for them there, which they would hate—"

"How do you know they would?"

"—which they would thoroughly hate, and would hate you for it, although you would expect them to be very grateful to you. And in ten years' time they would all be on welfare and you, my dear, would be complaining about paying their medical bills. No, let others with stronger stomachs than yours and mine go to India, and in their spare time pore over the ground plans and the plumbing systems of the medieval hospices (for it is all the same sort of chaos, and smells the same) and I will stay in my study with my favorite pipe and reread *The Decline and Fall of the Roman Empire.*"

Applause, and the company moves away from the table, into the living room with its splendid, panoramic view of San Francisco. The hostess brings coffee, and we sink into deep, leather chairs and velvet-covered sofa cushions. Somewhat to my surprise, I find that Professor N. has chosen to sit beside me.

"We were interrupted," he says cheerfully, "by an expert. A

very crafty flanking movement by the lady who has cherished me
these 40 years, though God knows why—and who never misses an
opportunity to remind me that we never travel. She does not
want to go to India at all, she wants to go to Paris. India was
merely a threat, a bargaining point. She knows me well. Now, tell
me about technology and the Hospice de Beaune."

"I will, thank you. But first, I want to say that I think you made
a very important point about gratitude, which is the downfall
again and again of the earnest liberal—who believes he does not
want it at all, though he craves nothing more than human
approbation—and who, when disappointed, is apt to become the
bitterest of all conservatives."

"She allows me to make a point now and then, in public. Of
course, I don't give a damn what anyone thinks of me. But she
will have her revenge, dear soul that she is, probably in the form
of a pregnant cat she has rescued from the pound by late
tomorrow, and installed at the foot of our bed. Marriage is a
marvelous institution, isn't it? I've never understood why people
needed anything else. Well, pray continue."

"My point really was that the care of the dying at a place such
as St. Christopher's is a great deal better because of scientific
advances than any that could be offered at Beaune in the fifteenth
century. The hospice at Beaune offered great cleanliness and
compassionate personal care, and spiritual guidance as well as
aesthetic grace. But I see two vastly important developments in
the modern concept, and one of them has to do with the relief of
pain. We know that opium poppies grew in the medicinal herb
gardens of St. Gall's in Switzerland as early as the seventh century
A.D. and we know that something similar to heroin, morphine, and
codeine—all derived from the poppy—was prescribed for severe
pain, along with wine and alcohol of course, in those days. And a
sort of polypharmacy was in operation, even if some of its
ingredients such as copper filings and the excrement of pigs
(sorry!) were not altogether helpful in the long run. And yet, we
have learned so much better how to mix and combine and
prescribe our medicines for pain relief, mainly because of the
work done in the modern English hospices. And we are learning
how to combine them with recently discovered mood-altering

drugs as well as other specifics so as to get maximum comfort for the patient. We have learned various nerve-blocking techniques and we do not weary ourselves any more—unless of course we are in an acute-care hospital—with such things as bleeding and leeching. We have the development of modern technology to thank for this pain relief, and of course, it should be used.

"Ahah!" says the Professor. "Now I have got you. Now I see that this passionate concern of yours is really about pain. It is the neurotic, if I may say so—yes, definitely—the neurotic and totally unrealistic modern fear of pain that is your hidden agenda. You are tenderhearted and sentimental about pain, which is, after all, one of the truly important ingredients of human life. Have you read Illich? Well, then. You say yourself that you admire the warrior, the one who embraces life. Show me the warrior who has never known pain and I will show you a coward. You speak of mood-altering drugs, but how does that differ in any significant respect from submitting to being controlled by the machine? Tell me that and I will listen gladly to anything else you may have to say about hospices."

I look at him and we both burst out laughing. "No, no," he says quickly. "I take that back. We have a long drive ahead of us, and we go to bed early."

"You are making two separate arguments here, I believe. One is about the necessity for pain and the other has to do with being controlled by technology. Well, then—but first, look at that view!" We are on a mountaintop and far beneath us, the city flings its lights across the lower hills. A plane passes over winking its own lights, red and green, against the starry sky, and below, scarved in long, fragile skeins of fog, the place that has been called "The Cool Gray City of Love" lies moving and breathing like a woman asleep, perfumed and dressed in all her jewels.

"It will not rain tonight," says the professor.

"No, I am afraid we shall have to wait for your Flood a while, and that in the meantime we shall have to do the best we can with human nature. Pain, I agree, is one of the important ingredients in our lives. But what is its importance, and what kind of pain are we talking about? Obviously, the pain of touching fire by mistake is useful in that it signals us to withdraw before we are badly hurt; and the lack of the pain reflex in a leper, for example, is one of the tragedies of the disease. But the pain of terminal cancer is not helpful in this way. Pain can be important spiritually, too. People who have not experienced any of that long-term, excruciating, and presumably hopeless pain—the kind that really annihilates us as human beings—do not know what they are talking about when they use the word *pain*. They are like a pilot in a plane looking down on the fire-bombing of Cologne and thinking it might be nice to toast marshmallows. I like the story about Einstein, who was approached by a philosopher who wanted to persuade him that pain was not real, that it was to be handled as a process of mind-over-matter. Einstein without a word struck him a tremendous blow, knocking him down, and then said, "Now, tell me what you were saying." So I agree that pain is in this way instructive. In fact, it might be a better world if all people who prescribe any sort of behavior for others had first experienced a good deal of it.

"However, the pain that too often comes with terminal illness is an utter waste. It does not serve to warn, or to instruct. Instead, it simply blots out, at one of the most important moments of our lives, all ability to perceive, to think sanely, or to be in any way master of the situation."

"Pain has an element of—what is it? Emily Dickinson, I believe," says the Professor, and continues quoting:

> Pain—has an Element of Blank—
> It cannot recollect
> When it begun—or if there were
> A time—when it was not—
>
> It has no Future—but itself—
> Its Infinite contain
> Its Past—enlightened to perceive
> New Periods—of Pain.

"Thank you. Yes. And of course, she could not have written that in the midst of the sort of pain I am talking about. She had to do it from memory. This is the kind of pain that has no past but itself; it is all present, and no future. The hospice cares for the future of the patient, and sees itself as a way station. This is why knocking a person out with morphine or heroin or whatever, in a hospice, simply will not serve. The opium den is no place for a pilgrim. Are you satisfied now that I am talking about the death as well as the life, in a hospice, of a warrior—in other words, that I am not being unrealistic, or even tenderhearted?"

"Indeed," he replies, "you are extraordinarily merciless. My own death is something I would far prefer not to know about. Give me some opium to put in my pipe when the time comes, and I will happily smoke it."

"I see. On the other hand, you do not approve of mood-altering drugs?"

"I approve of everything. It is you who are so particular. What is the difference between taking these drugs and letting oneself be controlled by all the technology and the machines you so deplore?"

"I did not make my point clear, then. Let me try again. What I mean is that human beings should not behave like machines, or think of themselves as a collection of machine parts developing squeaks and rattles, and therefore becoming useless, with the onset of a disease or of old age. It is the thought control of the machine that I deplore, the tendency we have to be brainwashed by them into believing that we are like them when we are not. Mood-altering drugs or mechanical procedures to provide relief from chronic, long-term pain should be available. But they must be administered by people who are wise as well as compassionate, so as to bring the consciousness of the suffering individual as nearly as possible to its normal, healthy state—not to produce false euphoria. I myself, for example, very much dislike the reasoning of some practitioners in the United States today who have been using LSD to produce 'religious' experience in the minds of the dying and thereby to 'reassure' them. Chemical euphoria is chemical euphoria, nothing more. And I do not think religious experience as an orgasm of the mind can be very authentic when artificially induced."

"A passionate concern," he says. "Yes, a passionate and an evangelical concern: *consciousness is all.* But you do not persuade me to go to a hospice myself or to support the concept, because I strongly suspect that you hospice people really want to tell me how I ought to go about dying, and that I won't have. No, I will die the way I want to die, thank you very much. Oh, I know what you are thinking. You are thinking, 'Good luck to you in the intensive care unit then, old boy'—but after all, perhaps it won't come to that. I may fool you. I may slip on a banana peel tomorrow morning and break my neck and there will be an end to it.' "

"He is always talking about this banana peel," explains his wife.

"Well, no," I reply, "that was not my thought. I was enjoying your determination to be independent, and thinking of General Grant. You rang very true just then, and you reminded me of a man I saw at St. Christopher's, sitting up sleeping in an armchair late at night with a bottle of port beside him, and a writing tablet on his knees. Which brings me, if you can bear it, to what I promise will be my final point about modern hospices and their improvement over the medieval model."

"Anything is bearable—as long as I don't have to go to Paris. I have been to Paris," he says.

"What I think of as the fully realized modern hospice, since having experienced it at St. Christopher's, you see, is not merely a medical situation, but a real community. People there are living as well as dying, learning as well as teaching, growing as individuals and as members of a team which is not organized on military or even on purely intellectual principles, but which has all the richness of a loving and a caring family life. Now this did not happen at such a place as Beaune—and does not happen at modern nursing homes—because they are specifically set up for the separate and reclusive care of the incurable patient, and the other members of a normal community are not present. To a certain extent, it was a feature of the monastic hospices, because the life in a medieval monastery tended to be quite rich and varied, and yet St. Christopher's has the advantage here of being ecumenical, open to all without respect to religious difference or indifference, and it is not cloistered or enclosed in the monastic sense."

"But you saw what happened at a place like the old Hôtel-Dieu in Paris!"

"This is why we need a great many more first-rate hospices. One place here and another there simply can't do it. Chaos would result if the admissions team at St. Christopher's did not grapple with it—sometimes very painfully—day by day. The integrity of the community is always at stake."

"Community," says the Professor, looking down his nose, "is a word that irritates me rather extremely. You seem very fond of it. I had some dreams of my own once, for a sort of group—artists, poets, that sort of thing—and saw it fall apart because of what people are. Community to me means rubbing elbows with a great many individuals I happen to consider peculiarly unattractive."

"You enjoy your friends a great deal, though, I notice."

"Well, of course, they enjoy me. Not everyone would. But I myself am not like most people, and I dislike the communal approach to life that tends to put everyone into a mold."

"The sort of community I mean does exactly the opposite, however—that is, it lets each person do things in his or her own way. It is possible to be communal without being communist; in fact, to me, the communist idea is appalling, like trying to make up a human body using nothing but feet, or nothing but hands. A monster results."

"Still, I am a private man, you see, and if I have not been cured of that by my wife, I assure you that no one else will succeed in doing it. She will help you with your hospices, I am sure, and she would probably love to go and work in one or be ill in one, if it came to that. I would rather shoot myself like an old horse and get it over with."

"Well, I am afraid I am being very persistent, but in that case, you of all people I can think of, very definitely need a hospice. I haven't talked at all tonight about the home-care programs that a hospice has, but one very important part of the hospice program is a plan to help anyone who wishes to, stay at home. If you should become desperately ill and beyond cure, a hospice team could help you to stay quite comfortably in your own study with your pipe and your slippers, and you could enjoy once more the downfall of Rome while preparing yourself to die in your own way."

"Who's dying?" says his wife, taking him tenderly by the arm and leaning against his shoulder. "It's time to go home. Nobody's dying. Look at that view! Doesn't it make you just want to take off and fly, all over the whole world?"

"It does not," says Professor N.

"I feel like an astronaut whenever I come up here. What space! Isn't it gorgeous? Look how tiny the city is down there, and yet there are all those people, and what do you suppose they are doing?"

"Murdering one another as usual," he says, "and drinking bad wine."

"Your husband has been very patient with me, Mrs. N.," I tell her. "Professor, I have enjoyed talking with you and I appreciate the challenge of your point of view."

"I think it was very interesting," says his wife. "And I think these hospices sound like a very good idea. So you must tell us more about them some time, and how to go about getting them started, and I hope we can have a whole lot of them in this country soon exactly like that St. Christopher's. And I will tell you one thing. No matter how long you live with a person and no matter how much you love them, one of you always has to die first and leave the other all alone, and that is terrible. I saw my own mother go through it and she was a wreck. She sat there for years afterwards and wouldn't do anything. I can't stand to be alone, I can't even stand to think about it. So I have made up my mind what I am going to do, when one of us dies: I am going straight to Paris."

New Haven

CHAPTER 9

In the course of the next decade, the Hospice program will
no longer be innovative, but will be folded right into the
existing health-care system. Everybody in the health field
will be sensitive to, and knowledgeable about, the care of
terminally ill patients and their families.
                    Dennis Rezendes, Hospice Inc., New Haven, Ct., 1976

I came up under such a dawn and with so tender a dying
crescent in the sky that I spent an hour in Paradise. What are
these days of glory? . . . I will hope that they are premoni-
tions, hints granted beforehand of a state to be attained. At
the worst, they are visions of such a state lying all about us,
the home of the Blessed . . . the supports of this life, and we
creep from one to another like travellers from inn to inn.
                    Hilaire Belloc

Driving on an unfamiliar highway behind the wheel of a
borrowed car is an experience which would have been identified,
one assumes, by early New England Puritans as religious. *Vide*,
for example, Increase Mather, 1674, *The Day of Trouble Is Near;*
Roger Williams, 1651, *The Bloody Tenent Yet More Bloody;* and
Jonathan Edwards, 1741, *Sinners In the Hands Of An Angry God.*
Yet the visitor pressing eastward through Connecticut in such
circumstances, early in the spring of 1977, manages to note with
pleasure, even so, the rainbow springing from dark snow clouds
ahead, and the swallows wheeling companionably above the
marshes outside the city, so gratefully named by English refugees

300 years ago, New Haven. At least one of the grim, Calvinist divines would have understood the deeper springs of this delight, for it was Edwards himself who wrote, one day when he was not entirely preoccupied with the Fiery Pit, "The beauty of the world consists wholly of sweet mutual consents, either within itself or with the supreme being," and who taught that, "bodies being but the shadows of beings, they must be so much the more charming as they shadow forth spiritual beauties." He too loved rainbows, as it turns out, and birds, and spiderwebs; and it is said that his wife, Sarah Pierrepont, was extremely fond of him, for one reason or another, as were their twelve children.

The offices of Hospice, Inc. in New Haven will not be hard to find today, we are told; temporarily they are lodged on the grounds of Albertus Magnus College in the residential district. But the modern pilgrim, plunging from the parkway into the thick of downtown, rush hour traffic is amazed, perhaps even more than the English may have been when they first landed on these shores. Coming as they did from a land so mild, finding themselves in a place of savage winters and summers brutally, tropically hot, with poisonous plants, snakes, and insects unknown to them, and among natives whose habits they could not understand, they banded together in the archetypal pattern of community, setting their backs against the wilderness and facing one another across a providential and sustaining central Green. Early New Haven had a homogeneity of purpose and manners, was intellectually and architecturally spare, tense, uncompromising, and austere. Somehow one expects it to be that way still, like the villages of childhood gilt-string bags, with their tiny blocks and stiff little trees only capable of being rearranged in a certain, limited number of combinations. But of course, it is not. New Haven today is a far richer stew, less pretty but far more startling and fascinating in its bizarre juxtapositions of different modes and styles of being. The slick highrises of corporate industry loom downtown beside the graceful and romantic, neo-Gothic spires of Yale; mouldering redbrick mansions of the nineteenth-century urban rich now serve as pocket ghettos crammed between, or are slapped with signs claiming them for art, research, commerce, or social service. Pale and prim, two-hundred-fifty-year-old saltboxes perch beside the wildest and most arrogant of Victorian fantasies which in turn abut new and oddly menacing structures of steel and colored glass. At the heart of the ancient village where sheep and cows once grazed, the green stands empty now, shaken on all four sides by heavy traffic and stared at by a row of eighteenth-century churches whose doors are locked, at most times of day and night, against twentieth-century crime. Waves of immigrants over the years have assaulted first the Indians' primeval ground, then the Puritan vision and structure of things, bringing with them the rhythms, the fragrances, and the social contracts of contrasting cultures—Mediterranean, Irish, Eastern and Central European, African—as well as the desperate need of refugees to take hold, to prosper and belong. The history of New Haven is to a remarkable degree the history in miniature of America itself; and so perhaps it is particularly appropriate that in this place of haven to so many, scarred and marked as it is by years of human struggle and suffering, the first modern hospice in the United States should have been born.

As we enter the city today, Governor Grasso of Connecticut is in the process of announcing her request to the State Legislature for $1.5 million toward the building of an inpatient unit for New Haven's hospice. Designed on principles set forth by St. Christopher's Hospice in London, the new facility will offer comfort and highly skilled medical care to the terminally ill from Greater New Haven and throughout the state, welcoming them in the pilgrim spirit which originally gave the city its name. The event represents a happy achievement, not only for Connecticut, but for hospice teams throughout the country who have worked long and hard in recent years to bring comfort and support to the dying in their homes. Now there will be a 44-bed facility for these patients, with hospice-trained nurses and physicians in attendance, and with a home-like atmosphere for families and friends of those whose needs for special care cannot be met in the home. It will prevent critically ill people from dying in pain, neglected or cared for by the unskilled; and at the same time, will prevent patients such as those with incurable cancer from being sent back

into the costly and (under the circumstances) inappropriate
systems of acute-care medicine. This gesture by the governor—
soon, quite evidently, to be ratified by the Legislature—will be
rewarding to citizens of Connecticut in many ways. Not only will
it offer the kind of attention realistically needed by patients and
their families at such a time, but it will provide substantial savings
in hard cash to individuals, to government, and to private
insurance companies.

Home care by New Haven's hospice has been shown to cost, on
the average, about $450 over a three-month period. This sum
would cover no more than a two-day visit by the patient to local
hospitals, where he could not hope any longer for cure, but would
necessarily be isolated during the final hours from familiar
surroundings and from usual sources of emotional and spiritual
support. At present, 68 percent of New Haven's hospice patients
are being enabled to die in peace and comfort in their homes, a
figure which concurs with the wishes of cancer patients surveyed
between 1969 and 1971 in south-central Connecticut. With the
addition of a suitable inpatient facility, economical because it
does not support the elaborate machinery of modern diagnostic
and aggressively curative treatment, the hospice will remove
from stricken families what is often a catastrophic burden of debt,
and will present to third-party reimbursement agencies, both
public and private, a service delivering substantial benefits to
them. Only 6½ percent of hospice patients in Connecticut can be
expected to be self-paying; the rest must rely on insurance funds.
Inpatient care at the new facility, when needed, will cost about
$100 per day, less than half of local hospital charges. The hospice
achievement is, in fact, a cause for general celebration. It is one of
the rare events in our time which is both fiscally creative and
morally sound.

The two-story building, white with red shutters (once a private
home), in which the Hospice, Inc. offices are now located is a hive
of activity today. Telephones are ringing, tea is brewing, type-
writers are tapping and jingling, it seems, in every room. It is the
sort of house, with unexpected stairways and odd rooms hidden
away at the back, that children love to explore; and there are

several of them here at the moment, as well as a baby in a basket in the front lobby, mingling with the nurses and the volunteers who hurry in and out, dressed in jeans, in business suits, in slacks and sweaters, picking up their assignments for the day. Several young women, nurses and social workers from the Royal Victoria Hospital in Montreal, sit chatting in the lobby waiting for the arrival of Dr. Sylvia Lack, Medical Director of the hospice; and I am taken in hand by Director of Public Information, Frank T. Kryza II, a tall, bearded young graduate of Yale, who spouts facts and figures as we race through the hallways, looking for a quiet place to sit down and talk. The mood here today is one of jubilation, for the governor has not only placed a seal of public approval on the nine-year effort of this hospice group, but has expressed her personal concern, breaking precedent this week, with the donation of an honorarium of her own directly to the hospice, rather than to the State's general funds. Fingers are crossed, but ground-breaking is planned for July, 1977. Three million dollars, Kryza tells me, has been the fund-raising goal for the inpatient unit. Hospice, Inc. has received about $500,000 for the purpose in private and corporate donations (and has had unusual success here, in reaching corporations); the rest of their funding must now come from a combination of state, federal, and private sources. Having operated for the past two and one-half years as a National Demonstration Center for the hospice concept under a National Cancer Institute (NCI) contract, they must begin in September to work on a fee-for-service basis, trusting that public concern for the project will eliminate resulting gaps in the budget. Will they survive?

It appears likely that they will. Executive Director Dennis Rezendes, an experienced administrator energetically devoted to the cause, tells me later in the day that insurance executives and legislators are beginning to discuss the necessity for some changes in the health-care reimbursement rules. The average hospice patient now is 59 (and will be younger, when those under 16 can be accepted), thus ineligible for Medicare; the average income is too high for Medicaid. But an exception has already been made by Medicare for patients under 65 suffering from kidney failure, despite the extraordinarily expensive and elaborate nature of their treatment by dialysis. It would seem both humane and economically reasonable to make an exception as well for hospice patients whose condition has been diagnosed as incurable, and whose life expectancy is 90 days or less. Rezendes points out that, under present legislation, people in this group are eligible for agency home care if provided for within two weeks since their discharge from a hospital, whereas most admissions to hospice home care are sought by patients and their physicians several weeks after discharge. Without a hospice, the only help available to most of these patients is back in the hospital.

Between meetings which will run until late tonight, and will begin again over the breakfast table, Rezendes thinks aloud, speaking very quickly, very directly, about the future of the hospice concept in America. His command of the subject is impressive; so is the sense that this very practical, earthy, and politically alert person has a goal firmly in mind which might, to weary cynics, seem purely utopian and visionary. It is not hard to agree with him when he says, "Look, it's happening. We're doing it. Our people have been working their tails off, to keep patients at home, and they're succeeding with 68 percent. That figure has gone up from 52 percent, just in the last year. But they've also shown us that we have got to have a backup unit. When the patient needs 24-hour care and constant supervision by physicians, it won't work otherwise. We thought at first we were going to need 22 more beds, but we have cut that back because of the incredible job our people have been doing in the homes. We're aiming for some cottages on the grounds, instead—places where couples or families can stay together temporarily and have our kind of total care, and still have their privacy. There are special circumstances, and also some people need privacy at a time like this more than others. We have to come to grips with that realistically. The wealthier people are, for example, the more they tend to be isolated even from members of their own families, and used to depending on hired help for their needs. I wondered at first whether people from the old families in the East would go for the hospice concept at all. Have you read Stewart Alsop's book (*Stay of Execution*, 1973)? That was beautiful. He convinced me. Here was a guy from that kind of background, and he has a great passage in that book, telling how glad he was to have the companionship of an ordinary, working-class man, a person he wouldn't have had much contact with under other circumstances, but here he was lying in the next bed, and they were both dying. . . . That was very powerful, very moving. We find hospices answering a real need for all kinds of people when they are in trouble, bringing them together and offering a real sense of cohesiveness in the society. We want to have a teaching center, too, for people who are going to be doing this all over the country, and that will be connected with us, but separate, because teaching and research are not going to take over here. Our job is taking care of the patient's needs, and the family. Anything else we do, fine, but that always comes first."

Public consciousness is ready for hospices now, he says; and advocates find encouragement in the flavor of the present administration in Washington, as well. In campaign speeches, President Carter has called for "effective and low-cost treatment methods" in medicine, avoiding the "duplication of expensive and underutilized equipment and services" and he has urged insurance companies to "write coverage in such a way that it does not stimulate the use of expensive medical procedures and hospital care when less expensive care will be responsive to patients' needs." By shifting the emphasis of care to the *patient's needs*, hospices provide exactly this sort of program; for when curative efforts have clearly failed and the time of death is near, what the patient needs is relief from pain and other distressing symptoms, plus freedom to live in the manner of his own choice during his final days and hours. He needs not to be abandoned or isolated from his usual sources of spiritual and emotional support; and he needs to know that he matters as a human being to those around him at this time. Hospices offer a creative response, as well, to the Administration's call for better preventive medicine. Studies here and in England, by Colin Murray Parkes and others, have shown that recently bereaved individuals are at far higher than average risk of developing physical disease, of having accidents, and of

developing behavioral difficulties which are destructive to the
public as well as themselves. The skilled counseling and the
support of a caring community provided by hospice groups can
go far to eliminate this problem.

Innovative programs can succeed, of course, only if they are
thoroughly understood and actively supported by the people. In
Connecticut, this seems to be the case with Hospice, Inc. Four
months ago a computer in Washington rejected the request of
New Haven's hospice group for $2.8 million of the two billion
authorized by Congress for essential Public Works Administration
projects including health facilities. This was to have been the
funding for the inpatient unit, but sidewalks and road renovation
to the tune of $6.8 million in the Hartford area alone were judged
by the machine to be more important. At this, the Commerce
Department was inundated by frantic and outraged communications from Connecticut citizens, begging them to turn off the
machine, use human sense instead, and "give us the facility the
computer cannot understand." The reply they received was
interesting. "We all agonized," said Assistant Secretary of
Commerce John W. Eden. "Of course, we all knew about Hospice
and we were hoping as much as you were hoping that Hospice
would be funded . . . 'Where's Hospice? Where's Hospice?'
everyone kept asking when the rankings of the various projects·
were being cranked out" (*The New Haven Register*, Jan. 20,
1977).

None of these nice, agonized people thought to kick the
computer, evidently, or to pull its plug out of the wall. So it won
that round, cranking out not only more and more sidewalks and
roads, but a $2 million garage for the city of Stamford, whose
local councilmen had voted repeatedly against the project. It took
personal intervention on the part of Governor Grasso, responding
to the obvious wishes and needs of the people of her state, to
counteract the mischief of the machine and to give a hearing,
instead, to human voices.

Having achieved the recognition and affirmation of government, Hospice, Inc. of New Haven has reached the fourth and
final phase of a process described as typical in our society by

George Rosen, in his comprehensive study, *A History of Public Health* (New York, 1958). The first move toward the solution of health-care problems is simply the recognition by an individual or by a small, influential group that a need exists, Rosen says. Second, local experiments—such as New Haven's Hospice, Inc., Hospice of Marin in California, and others—are undertaken through individual initiative, in an attempt to develop practical solutions. Third, an attempt is made by those participating to enlighten public opinion and to attract the attention of government; and finally, if the innovative model proves itself at that level, government action with affirmative legislation will ensue.

The growth of individual hospices in America to date, has followed this pattern precisely, and all over the country, the explosion of the hospice movement is suddenly conspicuous. Eight to ten years ago, hospices were hardly known outside the United Kingdom; two years ago, to the best of this writer's knowledge, only three teams in the United States were actively engaged in caring for patients on St. Christopher's cautious and demanding principles: New Haven, Hospice of Marin, and an interdisciplinary group operating well, but on a very limited basis, within St. Luke's Hospital in New York City. Today, the map in New Haven's cheerful sunlit lobby at 765 Prospect Street is decorated, one end to the other, with markers representing new hospice teams from Honolulu and Seattle to Maine, New Hampshire, Rhode Island, New Jersey and New York; from New York down the east coast to Pennsylvania, Virginia, Georgia and Florida; through the midwest via Ohio, Illinois and Michigan; west to Colorado and North Dakota, south to Texas, then clustered in California locations from San Diego all the way up the coast. The National Advisory Council, headed by Dr. Elisabeth Kübler-Ross, is made up of 124 community leaders and concerned citizens from states across the country. It is interesting to find so many hospice teams in California and in New York, for these tend to be launching places of sweeping social changes, but significant as well to find the program backed by such a wide variety of American communities all over the map. The fact that New Haven was a jump ahead, nine years ago, may be partly due

to the history and the nature of the city itself, partly to the
intellectual vigor of the university and the medical center in its
midst; but, as is usual in such cases, it is due in large measure to
plain, hard work by some extraordinarily perceptive individuals.

Reverend Edward F. Dobihal, Jr., Clinical Professor of Pastoral
Care, Yale Divinity School and Director of Religious Ministries at
the Yale-New Haven Hospital, was one of these; Florence S.
Wald, then Dean of Nursing at the university was another. Rev.
Dobihal had been concerned for some time about the care of the
terminally ill in his ministry, and the tendency of modern medical
practice to insist upon death-denying, dehumanizing procedures,
long past hope of cure. Florence Wald, in the late 1960s, began
collecting data on their thoughts and feelings from dying patients
in an attempt to delineate better their real needs—and discovered
that one of their needs was to be asked such questions by someone
who cared. When Dr. Saunders came to Yale (as she did several
times during the '60s) to show slides of St. Christopher's, and to
explain her methods of patient-care, Rev. Dobihal, Dean Wald,
and a number of others similarly concerned came together at her
forums and realized that they were all moving in the same
direction, toward an innovative model for the care of the dying: a
hospice such as St. Christopher's. Early participants came from
different backgrounds, different faiths and different disciplines
within the community. Founding board members of Hospice, Inc.
were Dr. Ira Goldenberg, a professor of surgery at Yale, Dr.
Morris Wessel, a New Haven pediatrician and writer, and
Katherine Klaus, RN, together with Rev. Dobihal and Dean
Wald. They were joined in early discussions by a psychiatrist, a
Roman Catholic priest, the director of a local nursing home, other
physicians, nurses, social workers, students, community leaders,
and members of the clergy, Protestant and Catholic, Christians
and Jews. Divided against itself as a city like New Haven now is,
in so many significant ways, it has nevertheless managed to find in
the hospice a place of "mutual consents" and of common concern,
rather like the plot of green that once served to nourish and
refresh the original pilgrims. To Jonathan Edwards, all this might

seem rather staggering at first glance, for he was not one to sit down and dine with a man from Rhode Island unless he was quite sure the fellow had been "saved" nearer home; but his own disquisition on the law of gravity might comfort him on this score. Sounding much like an earlier Teilhard de Chardin, in fact, he wrote of "the mutual tendency of all bodies to each other. One part of the universe is hereby made beneficial to another; the beauty, harmony, and order, regular progress, life and motion, and in short all the well-being of the whole frame depends on it. This is a type of love or charity in the spiritual world." Jonathan Edwards may not have been ecumenical, but he had an idea of how things hang together.

In his office at the Medical Center, I ask Rev. Ed Dobihal to comment, early the following day, on the spiritual aspect of New Haven's hospice group. "Our society is not really ecumenical even now," is his response. "Religious groups exist here side by side, but as separate groups. This has been an area of some tension for the hospice from the beginning, but I see it as a creative tension. Many of us—most, probably—have a religious motivation for what we are doing, but the way it is expressed is, in general, very low-key. I myself see the hospice as a place of ministry, and as a place for the consecration of death. But I can't have a satisfactory conversation about that with a man who has a pain in his gut and a wet bed at the time. We take care of the physical, the medical needs first. We do what needs to be done so a person can start feeling like a human being again. As a matter of fact, my wife Shirley, who is a hospice nurse, probably does more *ministering* in a sense to patients than I do. It was what I would call low-key at St. Christopher's, too. I went there daily when I was in London on sabbatical in 1969, observed, recorded opinions of 60-70 percent of the staff, and filled in for their chaplain. You might expect a difference, with church and state bound up in that society which is so much more homogeneous than ours, in any case. But I startled some of them, when I spoke to their group before leaving, by telling them that they had at St. Christopher's many of the important aspects of a church—the corporateness, the

congregational character, and the belonging, caring quality of
their operation. Some of them really hadn't thought of it that
way.

"Here we have people from very different groups, working
together, and I think one of the reasons we have such *esprit de
corps* even so, is that we haven't grown too large, we have those
elements of caring among ourselves very much at hand and
visible, though our expressions of it might not be the same down
to every last detail. We give each other space, and we don't lean
on patients for any kind of conversions, either. If they want to talk
about it fine; if they don't, that's their business. We let them know
we are available any time, that's all."

Rev. Dobihal sighs, throws his hands up, and makes a tragical-
comical face as he reminisces about the long struggle during the
1970s to establish New Haven's hospice. At first, he says, it was
committees and committees, meetings, research teams, and task
forces of all kinds. St. Christopher's, they were convinced, had the
finest model of hospice care available; their methods of operation
had to be learned thoroughly, and ways had to be found for
translation (pharmacological, psychological, financial) to the
American culture and idiom. Funding had to be found, community relations defined, and the need for a hospice clearly
established with local hospitals, medical groups, and social service
agencies as well as religious organizations. Hospice, Inc. became a
nonprofit corporation in 1971 with Dobihal as president; and he
later became Chairman of the Board as well. Grants were
received for studies and for education of the public from the New
Haven Foundation, the Sachem Foundation, the Van Ameringen
Foundation, the Kaiser Family Foundation, and the Common-
wealth Fund. Forums and educational events were held, the
media took notice, and volunteers turned up, many of them
professionals in the health-care fields; but it was not until 1973
when Dr. Cicely Saunders came again to New Haven, having
received by now an Honorary Doctorate of Science at Yale, that
the group felt prepared to begin looking after actual patients in
their homes. What they needed now was a hospice-trained person
to take on the tremendously demanding and challenging job of

being their first Medical Director. Casting about, they consulted Dr. Saunders, then watched a film she had brought to New Haven, showing a young physician working with patients at St. Christopher's. "How would you like to have Dr. Lack?" she asked. The New Haven group was impressed and excited—so much so, that a telephone call was made on the spot to London, and Dr. Sylvia Lack was persuaded to consider the position.

"They called and asked me," continues Sylvia Lack, taking up the story, " 'how would you like to come out to the States for a year?' It was ten days before I was to take up the job in geriatrics I had always wanted; but I agreed, on Dr. Saunders's recommendation, to talk to them, at least. Then I accepted their offer, not realizing at the time that there would not be patients to work with immediately." Another grant was necessary before the next step could be taken; and when the proposal to NCI was written, Dr. Lack carried it down to Washington herself. It is interesting to speculate on the first reactions of people at the National Cancer Institute, to the appearance of 31-year-old Sylvia Lack, accompanied by stacks of grant proposals for Hospice, Inc. Blonde, bright-eyed, and snub-nosed, she looks like somebody's nice kid sister who is president of the senior class and terribly good at lacrosse. But when she begins to speak, that image shifts, and the person who may have judged her on such a basis is likely to be left feeling more than a little abashed. Dr. Lack is a gentle person, not afraid (like so many British and Anglo-Americans) of emotion, but she delivers her message with unmistakably solid intellectual and professional clout. She has two voices, in fact, one very light, very young, and rather self-deprecating; and the other, deeper and firmer, the voice of someone who has experienced and comprehended a great deal, and who understands the uses of authority. "Sylvia Lack," several people have told me separately by now, "is our secret weapon." Having come into the community as a fresh face, a foreigner, a woman, and a person accustomed to taking responsibility in a society 22½ percent of whose physicians are female, she has been able to make herself heard and to win over many people to the hospice point of view who might otherwise have been uninterested or even, perhaps, antagonistic. In a male-oriented power structure, her appearance on the scene is comparatively unthreatening; and her crisp manner and her correct, British speech have undoubtedly been an advantage in Anglophile circles of New England society. Her public lectures often move people to tears, and to reaching for their checkbooks, or coming in to volunteer their services to the hospice, although she has "rebelled," she tells me, from such duty in recent months, finding that it interfered too much with her commitment to patient care, and to the support and development of the staff. Among the staff, in the words of Dennis Rezendes, "she has promoted an environment for the development of team spirit, partly because in her case, the usual genuflection that goes on between nurse and doctor doesn't take place. She is young, young-looking, and very brainy. She thinks on her feet, and she is extremely articulate."

"How do you manage here, with our democratic habits, after coming from a society which is so much more used to the hierarchical ordering of things?" I ask Dr. Lack as we pitch into a pair of large, rather damp hero sandwiches, at lunchtime in her hospice office. She herself has gone out for this provender, rather than sending a volunteer. "Well, of course, we are a team," she replies with a grin. "But I am kidded around a certain amount by staff here—was especially at first—when they sit around for hours muddling through some problem and then they turn to me, and they sigh, and say, 'Well, I guess it's time for one of Sylvia's *team decisions.*' I am in charge, I suppose, very much as Dr. Saunders is in charge at St. Christopher's, but we all work together and do what needs to be done."

"What kind of support system does your staff depend on? Psychiatric? Religious? Sense of community?" Not psychiatric, she replies. She has found the same thing true here that was demonstrated in a study at the Palliative Care Service in Montreal's Royal Victoria Hospital. The people who "stick" with hospice work are those (1) with some personal commitment to spiritual values, and (2) outgoing sorts who enjoy helping and caring for others. It is taxing work, and very definitely it isn't for everyone. At a recent meeting, she tells me, she was asked by a member of the general audience what provision was made at New Haven's Hospice for psychiatric counseling of the dying, and she replied perfectly seriously, "But of course, I don't consider dying a psychiatric disease," and, without any intention of doing so, brought the house down. Hospice, Inc., she adds, does have a regular psychiatric consultant, who meets with staff and volunteers once a week with an open agenda, and who is available for private consultation if desired.

The culture shock for Dr. Lack has been primarily a matter of finding herself in a society which does not have an old, commonly agreed-upon sense of mutual responsibility among its citizens. She finds it odd that Americans, resenting and fearing government control as they do, are willing to put up with a system in which their vital, medical needs are so thoroughly controlled by bureaucratic red tape. Compassionate physicians, she has noted, are apt to find themselves in the position of sending patients back to the hospital on somewhat invented grounds ("We'll just have to put an IV in her") simply because the insurance policy doesn't cover comparatively inexpensive home care of a far more appropriate kind. Hospice of New Haven has managed to keep the majority of its own patients comfortable at home with a variation of St. Christopher's medication known here as "Hospice Mix," and generally consisting of morphine in a cherry syrup with phenothiazine, taken at regular intervals and in dosages designed to block pain before it happens, and thus to remove the patient's anxiety about having pain build up. "We try to maintain an atmosphere of open communication with our patients. We do not press them to talk with us about death and dying but make it clear by our attitude that it is OK to do so. Denial may be a useful and appropriate defense mechanism. If the patient wants to move to greater awareness, we try to give the necessary space and freedom."

"How is it that you are in hospice work, Dr. Lack? Where did it all begin, for you?"

"India," she says. "I grew up there. My father was in business in Calcutta. I remember when I was very small, Mother Teresa's nuns used to come to the kitchen door begging. It was always an event, when they came, and I was given to understand that this was something important. They really believe, you see, that a person has no right to eat until after the others who are starving have been fed. Then, as a young girl, I worked one summer in an orphanage in the Himalayas." (Here she speaks for a few moments very quietly, carefully, about a Christian "conversion experience" and continues.) "So I was convinced, you see, that I must go to medical school. I planned to study ophthalmology; so many, many people in India are blind, for reasons that are simple to cure. I saw a doctor there with people lined up on the ground, dozens and dozens of them with only a matter of inches between, waiting for him to come and remove their cataracts. His assistants prepared them and then he came along, zip, zip, from one to the next. Then another assistant came and bandaged them up, and soon after that, people who hadn't been able to see for years and years could see perfectly. I thought that was absolutely fabulous. Then in England, during my internship, I found myself looking after the dying patients as interns generally did (the consultants were no longer interested) and I saw them put into the four beds at the very end of the long, long ward. And at Grand Rounds, the doctors would come along looking at everyone, but then they would stop just before they came to the last four beds, and turn back. I used to invent questions, anything to attract them to those patients who were dying, but they soon caught on to me. They would say, just before the end of the ward, 'Oh, Sylvia, would you mind. . . .' and send me off to do this or that, so as to get me out of the way.

"One patient in great distress there for nine months particularly moved me. She had a great deal of pain, complicated by family problems no one wanted to help her with. Inadequate medicines, not the right mix, and at the same time, the rest of her was not being taken care of. She loved gardening. I thought after she died, if only we could have responded to that, set up a little garden right there for her, all around her bed, what a difference it would have made. And that is the sort of thing, of course, a hospice *can* do. During my residency in ophthalmology, those were people who absorbed me—the elderly, and those whose sight was deteriorating. I was fascinated to see the strength in people adapting to stress or to aging, the power in people whose lives had totally changed, who had once been full of physical strength and now were totally unable to help themselves. Still, in such circumstances, they had such courage and grace. My basic question, of course, was, *what is a human being?* When I was at St. Bart's, they sent many of their dying people to St. Joseph's Hospice, so I found out about that. Then, after the year's residency, I worked part time at St. Joseph's, part at St. Christopher's, still intending to go into geriatrics. Just as I had the position I had wanted, they rang up from New Haven. As you can see, I am still here."

Very much here she is, and closely in touch, obviously, with all that goes on at Hospice, Inc. Having arrived unexpectedly, I find that my time is beautifully arranged for me by some magnetic power or other which seems, very often, to have emanated from the general direction of Dr. Lack's office. I am given, not only introductions and appointments, but photocopied directions for finding the homes of various people who, as it turns out, were exactly the ones I wanted to see (and who, as well, were without exception, people who wanted to talk). All this is done quite simply and I am not given an opportunity until after it is all over, to realize what a nuisance I must have been. Stopping for a moment in the lobby this afternoon to get my bearings, I find myself chatting with a group of volunteers who have come for "Family Lunch"—many of them bringing their children with them—and after hearing an outside speaker, have settled down for a sociable hour together.

Sue Cox, coordinator of this program, tells me that she now has a core group of 50 trained people, men and women of all ages, although the hospice has never actively recruited them; most have turned up as the result of educational forums, news stories or word of mouth. Nine are registered nurses and many more are LPN's, but all spend eight to ten hours of orientation with her, then do field work under the direction of hospice nurses before being given appropriate assignments. Nonskilled people serve in many essential capacities, freeing those who are skilled for more specialized nursing work; all are treated equally with one another and with professional staff. "Volunteers are respected here more than at any other agency I know," Sue Cox tells me, "and this is an important part of our team program. We review our work daily, then meet in a team conference every Tuesday which includes the social worker, the physicians, and all nursing staff. We cooperate with other agencies in the area and they respect us because of the high level of our medical intervention and our nursing skills, but they do wonder, I think, at all our *listening* to patients! And this is why we allow a great deal of latitude in the hours and times our people work. Fifteen of our people may not be working at all, during any calendar week (we have a waiting list of more than sixty, and we bring them in as necessary) but it is important for them to have time off, because in the case of the hospice volunteer the gift is so much greater—it is in a very real sense, the gift of one's self."

By the front door, a distinguished-looking middle-aged man in proper tweeds stands talking with a young, very Yale-looking boy of about 19. Student and professor, perhaps? Member of the board having a lunch-time visit with his son? Not quite; both of these, it turns out, are volunteers. The older man tells me that he was in business, is now retired. Heard Sylvia Lack speak at Brewster's house [Kingman Brewster, president of Yale] a while back, was fascinated. "Couldn't understand why they didn't pass the hat, then and there. Plenty of money in that room. Lots of people would have written sizable checks. Got to thinking about it, rather annoyed about it, in fact, so came round here to find the office and make a donation. Been here ever since, working as a volunteer. I do transportation, this and that. Talk to patients, mostly, listen to them. They like to have someone around who isn't in a hurry, and I quit being in a hurry the day I retired. I do this because I enjoy doing it."

"I've decided to go on to medical school now," chimes in the undergraduate. "We can't go on ignoring people who are dying just because we have become a death-denying society. That's got to change, and medicine has to change. We've all got to raise our consciousness. I didn't know what I wanted to do with the rest of my life until I worked here, but now, that's no problem."

"What's happening in our medical schools and hospitals these days?" asks Dr. Morris Wessel, Clinical Professor of Pediatrics at Yale University School of Medicine and a founding member of the New Haven hospice. "You walk in the door, you leave your humanity outside." We are seated in his living room, on a quiet street in New Haven, drinking tea. Dr. Wessel is a pediatrician of the sort who makes grownups wish they were small again and slightly sick with one of those ailments, like "growing pains," that kids don't get any more. He would come to the house, put a cold cloth on your head, and convince you in a minute, not only that there is order in the universe, but that the real cause of acne and bedwetting isn't what you feared. In fact, it is well known in New Haven that Dr. Wessel *does* make house calls, despite the fact that he is one of the busiest and most distinguished men in his field. "Why did physicians stop paying attention to the human side of the patient?" he asks. "Doctors sitting around the place impressing each other, talking about diseases, not human beings. I am tired of it, it makes me sad. How did this kind of ethos get established? Of course I refer my children with leukemia to the specialists, but I help take care of them, too. My colleagues often ask me, 'How can you stand being around the parents of a child who is dying, talking to them about the whole thing, and when the child is dead, having to take all the emotional outbursts?' They don't want to get involved. Why not? Of course it is painful, but how can you take care of a child without getting involved, without knowing and accepting the rest of the family the way they are? I take the flak, I *like* taking the flak, because I know it's helping and because that is what I am here for. That's what a doctor can offer at this tragic moment. He can accept the parents and other family members with their bitterness, and still convey the idea that he cares about them. Look, we need to have more GP's in this country, people who deal with medicine as a whole, who deal with families as a whole. We need to stop separating our professional functions into little niches in the hospitals and in the medical schools, in the office or home. Doctors and nurses need to see the results of their work; and the young doctors today need to understand that human beings die. It happens; that's reality. They should be rotated through a hospice on a regular basis, let them see firsthand what it's all about."

"Doctors can't do everything," says his wife, bringing a plate of cookies. "Sometimes I think we expect too much of them."

"I'm not blaming doctors," he says. "I am blaming the system, the ethos of it, the way medical education is being presented these days to the students coming along. It is so clearly said, if not by words, by actions, 'Look, if you're going to be a doctor, you'd better stop being human here and now.' The students who really care about their patients are often looked down upon. That's just crazy."

The telephone rings and the Wessel's teenage daughter, in bathrobe with hair newly washed, backs through the living room slowly, answering it, greeting the guest, continuing to talk then into the phone as she works her way toward the privacy of an adjoining room, with a cord of at least 75 feet following her; then she disappears. This moment, somehow so much a part of the warmth of this home and of the welcome I have received from hospice people in New Haven, stays in my mind long after. It is a "type," as Edwards might say, of *hospitality,* that ordering of things which allows each one of us to be a unique and separate individual within a group which is bound together, not by similarity, but by love. You walk in the door and you bring your humanity with you, when you work with hospice people; and this is true, whether you come as a physician, as a patient, as a volunteer, or as a nurse, or just as a visitor.

Gray trees, gray fields, gray sky, flurries of snow against the windshield; midstate Connecticut seems strangely empty and wan now as I drive north, arriving finally at what is now known as, a "planned community" in the midst of more gray trees, gray hills. Patti Ruot, LPN, one of the nurses who has been with New Haven's Hospice since its early beginnings, has just moved here with her young family. "What is a human being?" Sylvia Lack asked, tending the dying in London. In much the same frame of mind, I now wonder, "Can a community be planned?" It is centered, I see, around a park, and within smaller units, around spaces that will be green in the spring, and that can be shared. A good beginning, but can we come together in the geographical sense, for a grab bag of individual reasons, and then become transformed into a community? And if so, by what alchemy? The pressures of need and danger have been known to do it; many Americans, for example, discovered for the first time during the Depression, or during World War II, that they had neighbors. Must it be war or the equivalent of it in some crisis that brings us spiritually together? Or, is it possible that peaceable ways can be found, simply in the natural course of things?

"Sweet mutual consents" are certainly less likely than they might be, in a society which refuses to acknowledge the reality of death. Interdependency doesn't happen among people, each of whom believes that he is immortal in present form, so long as the medical factory keeps on supplying him with spare parts. The dark side of the Puritan mind was perhaps a necessary adjunct— the back of the coin—to that extraordinary, luminous vision of life in all its beauty and richness that we also find in the best of the early New England writers. Edwards saw the lilies of the fields and described the sounds of music with almost hallucinatory brilliance, filled with a sense of their fragile impermanence as matter, and their real, secret meanings as vibrations moving toward us from the world beyond death. In this, whatever we may think of his politics, he was as modern and as radical as our twentieth-century nuclear physicists, with their "charmed quarks"; and he would have no trouble at all understanding the radically spiritual dimensions of a modern hospice community. Hospice people today are all, in a sense, pilgrims and pioneers as he was, rejecting materialism and creating new dimensions in community life, even while they work with perceptions and ideas that are very old.

"It is a spiritual thing," Patti says of Hospice, Inc., "because it is a way of life, really. It isn't just a job. And I don't mean spiritual because of the clergy who are involved; I think there has been a lot of teaching *of* clergy here, as well as *by* them. But it is the feeling we have, of absolute commitment to each other, and to our patients in a different way from what you find in any other place. We are close to death all the time, and people ask me if that isn't depressing, but it really is not. Sad, but not depressing. The closer you are to it, the less you fear it. I feel like a daughter in the families where I've helped, or a sister. You know, when you are a nurse, you are supposed to be objective, do a job, not get involved, and look at your watch. We have to write down all the hours we work, the travel time, even the charting time, so the records can be kept straight, but it is very hard for us to remember to do that, in hospice work. Time isn't important. You do what is needed, and if a person needs you then and there, you simply don't leave. People don't stop dying at five o'clock. I've seen some beautiful things happen within our families."

Patti's son Brian, five, is dashing in and out as we talk, collecting mittens, reporting on the depth of the snow, and bouncing from time to time on the sofa beside his mother, while Melissa, 18 months, gurgles in her playpen, gnawing rubber toys. I ask Patti to describe the nursing system at Hospice, and she gives me facts, but this is not really what she wants to talk about. There are the equivalent of 62 nurses full-time on staff; they work rotating shifts and are on call. Patients can be referred by anyone, but must have clearance from their private physician to be accepted on our program. A nurse visits the family to do an assessment visit and if the family is admitted, she then becomes the family's primary care nurse, for continuity; someone must be in the home, either family or friend, to help; and the patient must be geographically near enough to New Haven for close supervision.

"Let me tell you about some of the great people I've taken care of," says Patti, having that over with. "There was a wonderful old lady who was so confused when we first went in, she thought she was in a nursing home. And she said, 'Look at this terrible, dirty place they have left me in,' but it was her own home. Well, we figured out what the matter was—mainly, just being lonely and having no one treat her like a social human being—and we got her on the right medicines and got her resocialized to the point where she used to sit up and watch TV with me and argue politics. She was really sharp. I'll never forget her.

"Then there was one family, they were Italian, and they had the old Grandpa right there in the kitchen with them while they were cooking, eating, laughing and talking and singing and he was part of the whole thing, while he was dying." Patti is nursing the baby now, and young Brian hurls himself onto her lap, thrashes around until he gets a hug, then settles on her knees. "Everything was going on all around him, and the last night I knew he wasn't going to make it, so I said I would stay. When we do that, it's called a 'bed-down visit.' It was time to wash him and his daughters helped me turn him over, but I thought I had better tell them he was so weak that even a little motion might stop his breathing, because I didn't want them to feel guilty about it if they were doing something when he died . . . Yes, Brian, he was dying, this very nice old man, and so I was taking care of him, that was the reason. Well, we did turn him, and he stopped for a minute, but then he started up again when we turned him back, very hard breathing (Cheyne-Stokesing is what they call that) so we knew the end was very close. I was so glad to see the daughters and the others weren't at all afraid. They were sorry, they were sad, of course, but they understood it was a perfectly natural thing. Having a chance when you are a family member to take care of the one who is dying is very important, I think. Then later in the night, he did stop breathing and he was dead. His two daughters just lay right down next to him, and hugged his body as if they were keeping him warm, and they cried, but they weren't afraid of the body, or of knowing that he was dead. That's the way it ought to happen.

"I am technically retired, temporarily that is, because once you really get into hospice work, you never retire, but I have to wait until the baby is a little older before I can go back, even to part-time work. It's such an ideal kind of work for me, because I can do it part time and still be really involved. It is so reassuring, too, knowing that the next person from the hospice is going to give your patient exactly the same care, and you don't have to worry about them the way you do in ordinary nursing. I go down for meetings in New Haven all the time now, as it is. I can't stay away. And I go to see my patients and some of the families of my former patients. You might say it is 'bereavement work' when I go to see the family, but we go through so much together, those people are like my own family to me, and I couldn't *not* go.

"I find the physical care of the person who is dying is the thing that helps them to feel close to you and really trusting. It is when we are giving a bath or a backrub, so often, that the patients suddenly want to confide. They tell us about all kinds of things, like one young mother who was so angry about dying, she was so young, why did it have to happen to her? She was upset about her body image, kept worrying about how unattractive she must be to her husband, wanted so much to live until her daughter graduated from school. I was able to share that, and give her some help with it because I was right in there with her in the situation, in the physical reality of what was happening. I wasn't just talking at her from some other place. People ask me, 'What do you say to them, Patti?' and I don't know how to answer that. I don't have any formulas, and I don't have any solutions really. It's just a matter of being as honest as I can and of really being there. One woman asked me, 'What's it like to die?' and she was crying and crying. I said 'I can't honestly tell you because I haven't died,' and I just hugged her for a long time, and we both cried. I have cried many times with my patients, but it doesn't give me a sense of being pulled down, but of being lifted up. Just feeling so much and sharing so much with them, it makes you know you are incredibly lucky to be there, and to be able to help in any little way." As Patti says, you have to be a hospice person; it isn't just a job.

"A hospice person" seems to be one who knows instinctively, whether or not the Latin root of the word is consciously perceived, that hospitality is the ability to be either host or guest, or both, and to find an equal sense of satisfaction in these two roles. As Henri Nouwen says, it is a matter of giving space, really—space in which people can be themselves. "Dying With

Dignity" is rather an unfortunate phrase, for what if a person isn't dignified by nature, or does not wish to give a dignified performance at such a time? Are we not *dignified* in the true sense, merely by being human: that is, *elevated* in some mysterious manner, not of our own doing, to the charmed condition of consciousness? Must we be pompous about it and continent, and keep our teeth in straight at all times as well? Contact with the living is, of itself, contact with life which is already in the process of dying; but contact with those who are about to make the final passage is a privilege not to be judged in ordinary terms. Against the dark, these lives blaze when given a little space, held tenderly; and the people fortunate enough to be truly present for the event are illumined by it.

It was a dying man, in fact, who in giving publicly the gift of self—though he had never until that moment been a public sort of person—may have done more than any stack of statistical arguments, or any of the perfectly healthy individuals involved, to tip the balance for New Haven's hospice when in 1976 they sought permission to build their inpatient unit in nearby Branford, Connecticut. The life and the death of Eugene Cote, U.S. Navy (retired), a quiet man, self-sufficient and independent by nature, will be remembered gratefully, as a result, by many who never knew him. Finding my way tonight over the parkway and down into the little town which is in so many ways still an eighteenth-century village, with crooked streets meandering and proudly floodlit, steepled churches, I see that I am, ten minutes away from New Haven's noise and bustle, suddenly in the heart of old New England, in a solid community very much aware of its past. Yet these are the people who led Connecticut into the fray, when the computer in Washington denied funds for a new and innovative model of health care in America; they bombarded the Commerce Department with angry protests and pleas for reconsideration of the project. The people of Branford know what the hospice can do, and they want to have it, not tucked away behind a hospital in downtown New Haven, but here in their midst, on a residential street and across from a public grammar school.

Eugene Cote's widow, Barbara, and their two teenage sons,

Michael and Robert, welcome me like an old friend into their
home: I have come to talk with them about Hospice, Inc., and to
hear the story of hospice care as they themselves, very directly,
have experienced it. At 9:00 P.M., Barbara has come from a
meeting of her choral group, tired, she says, but looking fresh and
energetic, a sturdy and attractive woman, blonde, expansive in
her gestures, and obviously loving, not only to sing, but to talk. "I
don't know what we would have done without the people from
the hospice," she begins, "I don't know how to tell you what it
was like, before they came. You see, he had a heart attack, and his
heart was bad, and then when they found his cancer—Michael,
Robert, when was it Daddy went to the hospital and had the
radiation treatment?—Yes, it was in 1973, and because of his
heart, they didn't dare operate. So he came home and he used to
lie on that couch right there where you are sitting, and it was
terrible. The pain was so bad, and he was a brave man, but if you
touched him even very lightly or if he had to move, he would
scream. The boys and their sister Patty were younger then, but
they would take turns staying up with him all night, every night,
trying to help him. He had chemotherapy, too, and it went on and
on, and then the people at the VA finally recommended the
hospice. We had heard of it, but we really didn't know what it
meant. They came right in, Dr. Lack came, and Patti was our
nurse. It was like the difference between night and day. It was a
whole new life beginning then, for all of us. They never made any
false claims. They said, we will help you all we can and we will
kill this pain for you—and they did. Gene started taking the
Hospice Mix every four hours at first and then he started feeling
so much better, he only had to take it every six hours. Finally it
was down to eight. For about a year then, it was absolutely
amazing, he was like his old self again. He was alert, he joked and
took an interest in everything, and he went uptown every day to
see all his pals at Jack's. I saw a real change in him then, in his
outlook on life. He had always kept to himself, but now he was
being so much more outgoing, looking at the other person's point
of view, being so much more responsive to those outside the
family circle. It was really wonderful to see him enjoying life that

way, taking it day by day, because, of course, we knew the cancer was in him, all that time.

"Well, the time came when the people from the hospice were here in our town before the planning and zoning commission and they were asking for approval so they could put their new building here. We went to that meeting, Gene and I. Some people didn't know what the hospice movement was about, and we heard some other people say it was gruesome, or sad to think about, and they didn't want it around. We heard and saw one architect explaining his plans, and it looked as if some people weren't really sure how they were going to vote on it. Then suddenly Gene stood up—I have never been so amazed in my life, because that wasn't like him, to push himself into the limelight—and he said, 'I am one of those terminally ill cancer patients the hospice is taking care of. . . .'" He actually said those words, *terminally ill.* Well, you could have heard a pin—you could have heard a *feather* drop in that room. Then he went on and told what it had meant in his own life, having their care, and when he was through, then I got up. I don't even remember what I said. I guess I told what kind of a change this meant for the rest of us, knowing we could count on those people 24 hours a day, any time we needed them. And you know one time, close to the end, I called them and said, I just can't handle it. I told the exchange I needed more help. They all wear those 'beepers' so you can reach them, and I hadn't turned around and walked up the stairs again before the telephone was ringing: 'What can we do for you?' It is the literal truth, there was an ambulance at our door 15 minutes later. Well, knowing that, having that to count on, it changes your life. The people at the VA were wonderful and I love them, they helped us a lot. But what a hospice does is just entirely different. Well, you know how the vote went, and thank God, because if there had been a hospice inpatient unit for Gene right at the end, it would have been so much easier.

"But they didn't have it built yet, so we had to go back to the hospital. You know, in the hospital, they take your medicines away and then they do a workup, that's the way they have to do it there. He was in such terrible pain then, that I couldn't stand it.

He had told me, sitting right there at the dining room table, that he didn't want any 'artificial life' when the time should come, and he had time then to teach me all the things I needed to know about insurance, and where the papers were, taxes, all that—what he wanted done—and believe me, that is important. But it is one thing to hear that in your own home when you are feeling safe, and another thing to bring it up in the hospital. Then he had a stroke, couldn't talk at all, and how could I be sure? The hospice nurses came right in to the hospital then and taught me how to communicate with him, asking him to squeeze my hand if he meant, 'Yes, I do want to go the way we have agreed.' I could see him trying so hard, so hard to squeeze my hand, and then he did. I knew it was right then, and the minister said I should respect his wishes; the doctors were good to us and didn't make him stay in the ICU any more. I sat with him at the end thinking about the good times, hoping he was remembering them too, like the trip we took that last year down the Blue Ridge Mountains. He was getting much weaker by then, and without the hospice, we never could have made it. And our 25th wedding anniversary, too, that same year—what a celebration we had. We wouldn't have had that, either. I have a lot to be thankful for, 25 good years.

"I was very tired when it was all over, I had trouble sleeping—me, having trouble sleeping, I couldn't believe it! And I kept getting sick, little things, colds one right after another. That was when I found out how much it means, not being dumped by the people who have been all through it with you. If I don't call up the hospice office, they call me pretty soon, or come around to see how I am. Patti and the rest of them are all like a part of this family now, and I love them in a way that is really something special."

We talk about the larger community around the Cote family now, Barbara's church, her many close friends and neighbors; she is an exuberantly warm and outgoing person who loves her job teaching in grammar school, enjoys all of her contacts in the community and is obviously loved devotedly in return. Yet, even under such circumstances, it has been all-important to her, that the hospice offered support and companionship at the deepest of levels, during the time of struggle and bereavement.

"How do you feel about having the hospice unit just across the street from the school?" I ask her.

"I think it's wonderful," she replies with enthusiasm. "They will be able to look out the window and see the children playing, and hear them going by. And the kids should be encouraged to get involved, too. Dying is part of life, and they should know it isn't something secret and awful, or something that has to be hidden. Hospice patients are comfortable and they are alert to such a degree that I can't think of a better way for young children to be introduced to this whole subject, than seeing them and mixing right into the same neighborhood with them."

It is hard to leave this pleasant home, even at such a late hour and knowing that I must leave Connecticut tomorrow. One does not merely "interview" people under such circumstances, and then go. The inquirer becomes part of the process, given such gifts of self, and is bound in to the organism of a hospice, both as host, and as guest. Was it a quirk of fate that hospice care gave to a certain man and a certain family in this town the time and the space for living in such a way that, at a crucial meeting, the gift so multiplied could be given back? Something called a quark, science now tells us, is the building block of all matter; we can't really find it, but we know it is there because it sends off minute, but tremendously significant, electrical charges. It would be interesting to introduce a quirk of fate to a charmed quark some-day, and find out whether they have any relation to one another besides the name. When scientists choose a word like "charm" to describe the melding behavior of atomic particles, they are obviously excited, a little nervous, perhaps, at finding anything so mysterious, but pleased; and one wonders whether next week's newspaper may bring the triumphant announcement of *"Physicists' Discovery:* Sweet Mutual Consents, etc, etc.—One Part of the Universe is Hereby Made Beneficial to Another." It would be entertaining if such a thing should happen, but perhaps not too surprising after all.

Walking down the corridor toward the closed door of the patient's room, being able to walk: it is a strange experience, powerfully illuminating and yet filled with mystery, each time it happens. The patient who cannot walk inhabits the same world as mine, but for him it is a world entirely different. Something will happen after I open the door; we have two hours to spend together, and during that time, in that space, I know our separate worlds will in some significant way become one. The process called "hospice" will happen; a melding, an interchange of roles and a shared glimpse outward, although there is no way for it to be forced, or even planned for ahead of time. It's a matter of something as mysterious as electricity. Like lightning you wait for it, and then you forget to wait for it. Then it happens.

The sign on the door says, *knock loud,* and so I do. An annoyed voice tells me to come in, and to shut the door behind me. I do that. Dark eyes, dark hair, a young, tanned body bare from the waist up, knees jackknifed on pillows, a thin, cotton blanket over him. A hospital bed, although this is a private home in a modest, residential tract. Trapeze above the bed, at arm's reach; also at arm's reach around the bed, books, stereo, CB radio, filing cabinets, plants, a small refrigerator, pictures, trophies, musical instruments, shelves packed with papers, notebooks, mementos. He appears to be about 25, angry. Very angry. Expecting me, of course, and now fully prepared to tell me a thing or two. We shake hands, I sit down, and we look at each other.

"The first thing you'd better know," he says, "is that I am not terminal. I am a very, very rare case, and I am an exception. I am not going to die. I have cancer, all right, but I am not licked and I have two different biopsies to prove they don't know what in hell is really the matter with me. What I need is for someone to pay attention to the fact that I am not like other people and do something about it, and I will talk to anyone and go anywhere and they can use me as a guinea pig if they want to but I want them to see that I am not a typical case at all, I am something else. It started in my back, I went to a chiropractor because I had this pain in my back and he just shifted it down lower. Then my van and I, we went to California, I had a good little rock group going and I was the manager—I used to be the drummer but I got pushed out of that because I was a better manager than the rest of them and California was good to me, but it gave me cancer. I found out I had it at UCLA. I went to the hospital there, and they told me I had a choice of—Hey, I'm going to tell you the whole thing and I want this on tape, why aren't you using tapes?"

"I'm sorry, I never use tapes with a patient."

"Why not? I'm not ashamed of anything, I've got nothing to hide, look, you can tell the whole world about me for all I care, maybe somebody will come up with a way to cure me then. Use my name. The guy from the newspaper already did a story on me, he used tapes."

"I guess I listen better without."

"Well, suit yourself but get it straight that I am not a quitter and I have not given up on this thing. I know how fast people lose interest in you in this world, when you're not fighting. They told me at UCLA I could have this operation where they would cut off my leg and cut a whole lot up around my hip, too, and if I didn't want to do that, then there was nothing else they had in mind. Well, I wasn't about to let them do that kind of shit on me so I told them, look, I'm going somewhere else. You say even that won't definitely cure me, why should I go for that? So I went to this place in Chicago, then to New York at Sloane-Kettering; I was in there for two weeks . . ."

Fast and furiously he goes on, telling of his pilgrimage, back and forth across the country in his van, which is parked now in front of the house, which he cannot drive any more. The disagreement of two doctors (he shows me the letters), the correspondence with the Mayo Clinic, the trips to Mexico, finally, smuggling Laetrile (no change that he noticed), then becoming weak, exhausted, having to come home.

"I'm independent," he says. "I'm a loner, always have been. Dad walked out on us when I was a little kid, and I was his oldest son. I changed my middle name that was the same as his, but it isn't any more. I don't need him. I don't need anybody. I am the kind of person, I don't owe anybody any money, they all owe me. Lying here like this—I've been flat on my back now four and a half weeks—is going to drive me nuts, and I am trying to control my diet so I get plenty of protein and vitamins and good stuff, but it costs, and that is really hard on the rest of the family." He pauses, lights up a thin, small cigar and takes a long look at me in silence. Finally, he says, "You want to see it?"

"Yes, if you don't mind."

"I don't mind. Have a look." He pulls the blanket down toward his knees. It is a very large, rather pale swelling all around the area of his left hip, firm and smooth to the touch.

"Are you in pain?" I ask.

"Not now, but I will be. Later. The pain now is in my head, thinking how maybe there is a way to cure this, and it's just nobody knows, and by the time they find out, it will be too late. Some doctor in New York was going to do this radiowave treatment on me and I thought a month ago that was going to be it, they would just get that thing going and melt it all down and then I would shit it out of me, if that's the way you get rid of cancer. They carried me on a stretcher down to New York, my friends did, but when I got there this man just said they weren't going to try it on me after all. He was really cold about it too, just said, no. Not that I blame him, somebody probably just put him up to it and he had to be the one to say it, but that was a really bad moment for me. I can't play drums any more. I used to be a really good drummer, we had a good little group. I tried bongos, but I couldn't do that either. Then I thought, maybe I could take up the guitar. I'm just too tired. No, I don't mean tired now, and don't try to help me fix the blankets because you don't know the right way to do it, and I will just have to do it all over again. You know Dr. Lack? I like her a lot. Yeah, these hospice people, they're all right, they don't try and fake you out on anything and they don't lay any trips on you, but that don't mean I'm giving up. That'll be the day, when I give up. My grandfather, he died of cancer and he never said a thing about it to my grandmother, she just found out at the very end when she saw, you know, the blood. I try to keep myself in shape.

"Look at my chart," he says, lying back, slowing down a little now, closing his eyes from time to time. "It's all there. Dr. Lack came over a couple of weeks ago and I got started with that stuff she gives. Before that I was popping methadone by the handfuls and it wasn't doing one damn bit of good. I give myself shots now, they taught me how, but I hate to stick myself with a needle and I hate any kind of drugs, I saw too much of that when I was in the rock scene, people on hard stuff, wrecking their lives, blowing their minds out; I smoke some in the afternoon—marijuana, I mean—because it helps me to keep up my appetite and I have got to keep that up. Look, you want to see the pipes I made? I carved them myself, I used to sell them. Over there is a picture of me, I'll bet you don't recognize me, that was two years ago. I was in pretty good shape then. Now I really think I am getting tired."

"I'm going in just a minute."

"Did you see that trophy? That was for being the CB operator that came from farthest away—no, up there, on top of the refrigerator, you're looking the wrong way, turn around—that was when we all got together and I was the one who came from the farthest. I always did like to win. I've traveled a lot. There was a girl—well, there were a lot of girls, but not too many. I traveled a lot, I kept moving. I guess I've been almost everywhere in the good old USA there is to go, now that I can't go anyplace any more. I see you notice that crucifix over my bed, well that doesn't mean I am religious, that just means, someone put it there. I went to catechism a few times, then I cut out and didn't go, so the priest came and said if I just came for the last lesson, they would let me be confirmed, and I thought, what kind of a deal is that, it can't be worth much if it's that easy, if they want you that bad to get into it, so I said, no thanks. So I am not religious. I don't believe in all that hell and punishment kind of stuff either." He is speaking very slowly now, with eyes closed. The little room is very close, the air is dense. He kicks at the end of his blanket, I try again to help him with it, he looks at me and smiles. "When I die," he says, "I am going to be cremated. Or maybe I shouldn't do that, maybe I should donate my body instead so they can figure out what the diagnosis was. But then, even if they find out, I will never know, will I?"

"Maybe you will."

"Maybe I'll be reincarnated and come back as a dog or something, that would be funny, wouldn't it," he says, unsmiling.

"No, not a dog. You're a drummer." We both laugh. I am putting on my coat. His eyes are very tired now, he puts one hand up to his forehead, touching himself as if asking a question with his fingertips.

"You are going to California tonight?"

"Yes. I wish I didn't have to, but I must."

"Say hello to California for me," he says.

"I will."

We say a few more words. Ridiculous, shaking hands, telling each other that we will keep in touch. "Thanks so much," I tell him. Then, standing by the door, having forgotten by now long ago about rainbows and quarks, about charm and vibrations, lightning and lilies of the field, I suddenly hear him speak to me in a voice so tender and gentle, it is like the voice of a lover, or of a mother speaking in private to her child.

"Take care," he says. "You have a long way to go, and it's hard, traveling alone."

A Matter of Depth

CHAPTER 10

The old order changeth, yielding place to new,
And God fulfills himself in many ways,
Lest one good custom should corrupt the world. . . .
But now farewell. I am going a long way . . .
To the island-valley of Avilion;
Where falls not hail, or rain, or any snow,
Nor ever wind blows loudly; but it lies
Deep-meadow'd, happy, fair with orchard lawns
And bowery hollows crown'd with summer sea,
Where I will heal me of my grievous wound.

Alfred Lord Tennyson

In ancient Welsh mythology, Paradise was *Ynys yr Afallon,*
which in translation is, "The Isle of Apples," or Avalon; and it
was to that magic island that the black-draped barge brought
King Arthur, mortally wounded, after the last battle of the
Knights of the Round Table. Avalon was the kingdom of the dead,
and yet at the same time it was a healing place, happy and fair
with orchard lawns, and if in those orchards apples grew, they
were a symbol from times long before the beginnings of Arthurian
legend, of fertility, natural renewal, and human love. Arthur had
seen the end of his noble dream of a community pledged to the
highest of chivalric ideals; destroyed from within, the old order
failed after its brief flowering at Camelot. He himself was near
death—and the historical Arthur, a military chieftain and cavalry-
man, may have been buried at Glastonbury in the west of
England long ago—and yet, in the minds of the poets who sang his

story, his ultimate destiny was one of mystery, in which dying itself was seen as a journey toward the island where he would be healed.

From Devon and Cornwall in the West, those lands of mist and starlight, soaked through with centuries of Arthurian legend, came many of the tough, seafaring Yankees who first settled on America's northeastern shores. Some of our early colonists were chivalric; but many of them, unfortunately, entertained, about the "New Jerusalem" they planned to found in the wilderness, ideas which were anything but high-minded, noble, or kind. Survival of the fittest, though it was not a familiar phrase then, was a rule invested in early New England with all sorts of self-righteousness and piety. The poor widow and the helpless orphan were not subjects for gallant rescue and celebration here; they were social misfits, and if they were ill, as well as useless, then many of their neighbors were ready to assume that it was their own fault. Good health and material prosperity were, in the eyes of second- and third-generation Puritan immigrants, a sure sign of heaven's favor. Poverty, illness, and other forms of social impotence were proofs of sin, and of punishment by the wrathful Jehovah they invited to preside over their narrow and obsessive, almost paranoid, readings of the Old Testatment. When plague and pestilence struck, "God's Controversy With New England" by Michael Wigglesworth (1662) expressed the attitude typical of the day:

> One wave another followeth,
> And one disease begins
> Before another cease, because
> We turn not from our sins.

The idea of quarantine (literally, forty days of isolation) for contagious diseases was by now a very old one and was practiced, particularly in the seaports of the western world, as a practical measure for the promotion of public health. "Foul vapors," "boggy places" and such were generally thought to cause disease, and germs were not yet understood, but it was common custom to separate victims of ailments like plague or smallpox, when possible, from the rest of society. To this separation and quarantine our early colonists could not help adding, because of their religious beliefs, a sense of moral rebuke. Foul sins, they thought, must have caused their neighbors to fall ill in this new land so pure and clean (as it was then), and the agony of disease and the shame of death were their punishment.

Under the circumstances, it is not hard to imagine the feelings of such a person as the Widow Paige of Boston when, on June 20, 1702, selectmen of the little town discovered that she and her family were suffering from smallpox. A warrant was issued, soldiers came to her door—perhaps she had time and energy to gather up a few personal possessions if she had any, or food and bandages to bring with her—and the family was loaded into a boat and banished forthwith. Had she tried to hide herself away, one wonders, kept the children behind curtained windows while she heard echoing in her ears the terrible sermons of the day about the fate that awaited her, burning until the end of time in the Fiery Pit? Had she bargained with God by candlelight for the life of her youngest who, though "born in sin," had surely not yet learned to practice even the smallest cruelties of the day? Was she a widow because her husband had already died of the disease, and if so, should she have nursed him in his loathesomeness, or abandoned him to heaven's wrath? How strange it is, knowing what we do about the deeper meanings of the name, to find in the old public health records of Boston that the place of isolation chosen for Widow Paige was a nearby spot called Apple Island. There, in the warm June sun with clear saltwater to bathe their ravaged bodies in; with fish to catch, clams to dig, wild fruits, herbs, and the air around them as yet unpolluted with cancer-producing chemicals, perhaps the widow and her family managed to recover, if not their moral credibility, at least some measure of physical health. But whether they lived or died on Apple Island, surely some inner healing must have resulted from their stay. It was sanctuary for such a group, merely to be removed from the suspicion and the contempt of their former neighbors. And islands by their very nature, as all travelers know, have a way of luring the human mind out of old habits, sending it on farther and freer journeys.

Most sick people, of course, in the early colonies, were cared for at home by women who had learned at their mother's knees the ancient lore of herbal medicine, growing these "simples" in their kitchen gardens and adding to this heritage whatever could be learned from local Indians. The trick was to do it well enough to survive, and to help your family and your neighbors survive, without being taken for a witch. Until the mid-eighteenth century, American families were expected to care for their own, or if afflicted with something contagious, to repair to some makeshift hospital or "lazar-house" which was apt to be a military fort with soldiers standing guard. The first general hospital for the care of ordinary citizens was founded in Philadelphia in 1751 under the auspices of Benjamin Franklin, who vastly enjoyed the political sleight-of-hand he employed in getting people to open their purses for it. Seeing that there was not enough money available, either in the public treasury or in donations from the rich, Franklin invented on the spot the device so often repeated since, and so peculiarly American, of "matching funds." Thus began the tradition of medical philanthropy which has continued to this day in the U.S.A.: one part practical benevolence and another consisting of a profound dislike for, and suspicion of, government control.

Incurable patients and those with contagious diseases were specifically excluded from this and other early "voluntary" hospitals in America, and a great deal of fuss was made over the distinction between the "deserving poor" who could not receive proper care at home and those judged "undeserving" of hospital care on moral grounds. It is interesting to find that the stated reason at the time for a public hospital to be built in Philadelphia was that, by now, too many strangers were wandering about town with no one to look after them when they were hurt or sick. The situation harks back to the opening of Fabiola's place of hospitality in the first century A.D., and to the tradition whereby pilgrims were welcomed, sick or well, in the medieval monasteries. Ben Franklin was himself a devout Christian, though he evidently bent the rules a bit whenever he had an opportunity to go to Paris; but he was also a wily politician and a supremely practical man. He chose exactly the right sprinkling of theological persuasion to sweeten his fund-raising appeals, reminding his fellow Yankees that these sick strangers "may possibly one Day make part of the blessed Company above, when a Cup of cold water given to them will not be unrewarded." If he had suggested bread and wine, fine linen, and silver goblets (which were given to the sick by Hospitaller Knights in the eleventh century, while they themselves subsisted on plainer fare) one wonders what might have happened. As it was, the image of Lazarus at the gates prevailed, well buttressed by a system of moral judgments and political-economic checks and balances; Franklin's campaign was a great success.

And so it was with mixed motives and mixed feelings, that our American system of hospital care for the sick came into being. Part fortress, part place of refuge for the "respectable" poor and for strangers who looked as though they might be useful some day, the American hospital has been, above all, a pragmatic response to health-care problems in the society. During the nineteenth century, special hospitals for particular conditions appeared; and notions of hygiene improved to the degree that people with contagious diseases were now received into the general hospital for palliative care and, if possible, for cure. With the tremendous scientific advances of the past century, and the growth of research and teaching centers connected with our great, modern hospitals, American medicine has come to serve people at every level of society in ways that could not have been dreamed of by the early settlers. Meantime, American medicine has entered the arena of big business and has done very well there, although it should be noted that in 1973 Americans spent more on tobacco products than the pretax net income of all our physicians, and $3 billion more on alcoholic beverages than the gross income of all American physicians combined.

Not to be put into the same ward with the Widow Paige, when we have come into the hospital for open-heart surgery or merely with a broken leg—this is part of what we pay for when we deliver our bodies to the modern medical factory today. We expect and demand hygienic conditions, and despite the continuing problem of infection (which is not new, although it has received a good deal of public notice of late) within this system, standards of protection in American hospitals are probably the highest in the world today. So are the prices we pay. In financial terms, it is generally agreed that this cost is outlandish, catastrophic, and not to be borne any longer; the crisis in medical management in fact centers upon the day-by-day price of hospitalization in a system which represents an effective monopoly on the market. We pay a cost for hospital services in human terms as well. Upon entering these walls we surrender ourselves to be held in a curiously prison-like sort of detention, incarcerated while ill or injured as if being punished for some crime. The old, Puritan attitude of moral rebuke is now unspoken, unrecognized perhaps; but it is there, nevertheless, in the condescending way we are treated, in the way in which we are stripped, numbered, and handled, given isolation without privacy, and sterility without the sort of cleanliness that is refreshing to the soul. If we fail to be cured and are dying, we become true pariahs in this environment. Being sick is no longer consciously felt, by most twentieth-century Americans, as proof that we have sinned against God. Nevertheless, we are treated like sinners in most hospitals, and if we slip lower yet and refuse to be healed by the "miracles of modern medicine," we become exiles from grace, banished within the establishment to a far worse place than Apple Island.

This is not to say that the hygienic standards of our hospitals should be relaxed in any way. Quite the opposite, in fact; with the delicate new procedures now being undertaken, the organ transplants and the explorations by scalpel into brain and heart, sterile conditions in the acute-care institutions must be zealously guarded and continually improved. However, 67 percent of deaths in America today are the result of heart malfunction and cancer: two noncontagious conditions which demand expert medical and nursing care without requiring the patient to be put, for the protection of the rest of society, into quarantine. Elderly people suffering from noncommunicable ailments now occupy no less than one-third of our hospital beds, and many of them, because of their weakened condition, fall prey to the sorts of infections that develop as often, or even more often, in the hospital than at home. Very few people are now sent to hospitals for rest or convalescence, or if they should be admitted for such a purpose, would find it a restful experience. Yet we ship off our dying to hospitals quite automatically, simply because they are dying, and we assume that this is what we ought to do. In the case of cancer patients in the terminal stages it may be that we have tended to become particularly panicky on this score because of the old superstition, still dying hard among people who are otherwise quite well educated, that cancer is a contagious disease. *But cancer is not contagious.* That much about it, we do know.

Our reasons for rushing off to the hospital with our dying cancer patients are not so simple as the fact that we are afraid of cancer, afraid of death, and do not want to watch what happens when a person dies. Medical history in America has woven a web of circumstance around us lately, which leaves us feeling unable to assume personal responsibility in the matter. In the "good old days" the family doctor or GP was available to come into the home daily, to help the patient remain as comfortable as possible there with regular doses of powerful opiates, and to participate in the process, both as physician and friend, of sickness, death, and mourning within the family. At present this sort of physician is so rare in our society as to be nearly extinct; and not because American doctors have all become suddenly lazy or disinterested. An entire book could be, and perhaps should be, written to explain the disappearance of this species. Some immediately obvious reasons are, first of all, the difficulty of achieving and maintaining sufficient medical expertise as a GP in an era of expanding information such as the profession has never known; and the ever-increasing tendency of the American people to rely on specialists, and to pay their far higher fees, for the simplest of diseases. "What's the matter with you doctors nowadays?" an angry man remarked to his wife's general practitioner recently. "I can fix any machine in my house, but I have to go to ten different doctors downtown when my wife gets sick, and none of them can fix her." The GP had been trying, in the kindest way he knew, for some months to help this man understand that his wife had cancer, that it was inoperable, and that she was dying. Meantime the specialists were responding, one by one, to the man's view of his wife as a machine with a broken part somewhere, and were collecting their fees; and the GP, with a wife and a family of his own to support, was in debt.

There are other reasons, as well, for the disappearance of the family doctor and his traditional house calls. As early as 1899 in New York City, the corporate power of hospitals, clinics, and dispensaries was beginning to be felt as a threat to the successful continuance of this kind of medical practice. Rich as well as poor people developed the habit of turning to the institution, rather than the individual, for medical aid; and in the meantime, sensational new procedures within the hospitals multiplied so rapidly that these structures became shrines in the public mind, places of magic that could defeat, it was supposed, even the power of death. Because of the disappearance of various contagious diseases such as typhoid fever and diphtheria, together with the decline in infant and maternal mortality rates, life expectancy for the average American soared, between 1900 and the present, from 47 years to 70. Wishful thinking made it seem that this curve, like a rise in the stock market, would go on forever, even though after 1929 we perhaps should have known better. Several generations of Americans by now, accustomed to using the emergency room at the local hospital as their personal physician, believing in the mystique of those shining fortress walls, have grown up without ever having had the experience of death and dying in the home, and without having any sense of its being appropriate. What was not seen, no longer heard and participated in as a normal event was now whispered about, feared and finally, ignored or repressed.

The situation itself is a sick one, and in seeking to heal it, the modern American hospice reaches back to retrieve what has been most humane and sensible in our own medical history, and beyond that, to a time before we believed that we must be invincible in order to win the approval of God. At the same time, the hospice movement thrusts toward the future in its development of finer techniques for therapeutic and palliative care, and in its enlightening concepts of personal value and of human community.

The hospice, obviously, is an idea whose time has come in our culture. For this reason, it is important that its characteristics should be clearly understood by the general public as well as the professionals involved. Here we are not dealing with a casual fad or a matter of fashion. Instead, we are dealing—quite literally— with matters of life and death, and with moral issues that will affect every one of us, directly or indirectly, as time goes on. The history and the philosophy of hospice care are closely intertwined; and it is possible to understand a great deal about both simply by being present in a hospice such as St. Christopher's, or by working with the people of Hospice, Inc. in New Haven, and Hospice of Marin. More is needed, however, if we are to have available for ourselves, our friends, and our families, the kind of care we can trust. Standards must be set, and defined down to the smallest detail. As we all know, an idea whose time has come is, per se, one extremely vulnerable to exploitation and abuse. This must not happen in a matter so serious as the care of the terminally ill.

The United States Government has recently prepared a description of a hospice which, though brief and therefore necessarily incomplete, serves as an introductory definition:

> HOSPICE: A program which provides palliative and supportive care for terminally ill patients and their families, either directly or on a consulting basis with the patient's physician or another county agency such as a visiting nurse association. Originally a medieval name for a way station for pilgrims and travellers where they could be replenished, refreshed, and cared for; used here for an organized program of care for people going through life's last station. The whole family is considered the unit of care and care extends through the mourning process. Emphasis is placed on symptom control

and preparation for and support before and after death, full scope health services being provided by an organized inter-disciplinary team available on a 24-hours-a-day, 7-days-a-week basis. Hospices originated in England (where there are about 25) and are now appearing in the United States.

> (From *A Discursive Dictionary of Health Care,* prepared by the subcommittee on Health and the Environment of the U.S. House of Representatives.)

Beyond this, qualifications for authentic hospice care are in need of more explicit inspection and definition. Before moving on to a study of several rather different hospices models in England, Canada and the United States, it may be useful to summarize here what has been learned thus far. What, let us ask, does the word *hospice* in the twentieth century mean?

First and foremost, a hospice is a caring community. This does not mean a group of well-intentioned people who want to be helpful to others in some vague way; and it does not mean a group serving any "special interest" in political or economic terms. It means, a group of people who are growing (or have grown) into a community by means of their shared dedication to a particular task: promoting the physical, emotional, and spiritual well-being of the dying and their families. In the process of hard work at this task, of sharing their skills and sharing themselves with one another, they become a community of people who care, each for the other and all for the people they serve. The diagram of a community is a circle with a center. At the center of the hospice community is always one thing: a body coexisting with a belief. The body is the dying patient's; and the belief is that the patient is something more than his body.

To the Christian, the patient's body is, quite literally, the body of Christ. To the Jew, the patient may be the angelic messenger who in ancient scripture was welcomed and refreshed, by God's command, in the form of a human stranger. Moslems, Hindus, and members of other faiths have similar beliefs; so do compassionate people who prefer to call themselves merely humanists. It is not necessary for a person to belong to any formal congregation or religious group in order to become a valuable member of the hospice community. What is necessary, however, is a sense of the mystery and the spiritual dimension of life. True caring and true community do not happen among people who think of one another as functional units in a system designed for efficiency. This is why hospices cannot be constructed by systems analysts on paper, and then be made automatically to work. Hospices cannot be understood by computers (though, like human beings, they can make good use of them) and they cannot be legislated into existence (though, like people, they may need some measure of sensitive legislation to protect and to guide them). People who come into hospice work without being suited to it, or who fail to understand it, generally tire of it rather quickly and drop out. In this way, the hospice community is quite efficient as a self-pruning organism with its own destiny.

Second, a hospice is a community of people who are highly trained in their various skills, particularly in the art and craft of medicine. The medical staff must be expert, not only in conventional disciplines, but in the newer methods of pain control and symptom control taught at St. Christopher's. Psychiatrists and pharmacologists working with the group must be fully qualified; nurses must be experienced and competent as well as sympathetic. A hospice must provide 24-hour-a-day, 7-days-a-week availability of medical and nursing staff for any patient and family it accepts. A group of "caring people" no matter how well-intentioned they may be, cannot pretend to be a hospice unless they practice hard medicine of this sort, and have the staff to provide it in whatever measures it may be needed. Faith-healing groups and prayer groups, though they may be able to accomplish many good things, are not hospices. Groups or individuals promising to provide "an easy death" by removing the patient from medical professionals and performing some sort of hocus-pocus with or without the use of drugs are so far from being hospices that it is hard to imagine them trying to use the name; but there are reasons to believe that some will, and they should be guarded against.

Third, the hospice offers its services and its fellowship, not only to the patient, but to the entire family unit. These services are practical in every possible way, from transportation to aid with planning finances or making a will; they are also psychologically effective in that trained therapists are on the job to notice difficulties, practice preventive medicine where possible, and offer guidance to any family member who wishes it. Close attention to the spiritual well-being of patient and family is an integral part of hospice care, with clergy and lay people of various denominations available to provide companionship at the spiritual level and to perform whatever rituals may be appropriate. The hospice community embraces patient, family, and close friends, not only during the final days and weeks of the patient's life, but long after death, offering consolation and support during the time of bereavement.

Fourth, the hospice cares for as many patient-family units as staff and volunteer support will allow, without distinction between any on the basis of race, color, creed, or ability to pay. Different hospices have different sources for their financial operation; most depend on more than one source, and payment for services is acceptable from the family that can afford it. But empire-building is not the appropriate motive for a hospice; therefore it is a nonprofit organization and whether public or private funds are used (or both) its books must be open for inspection by the larger community at all times.

Fifth, the hospice is a community operating on its own principles, which are not the principles of a hospital or a nursing home; therefore, the hospice must be autonomous in terms of its professional procedure. Legislation as it may be needed will perform the service of recognizing standards of care which are already being practiced at St. Christopher's and its closest followers in Britain and America; but different hospices are developing slightly different forms of operation, reflecting the nature of their various backgrounds and neighborhoods, and this should be taken into account. A hospital is not a hospice, and cannot become one merely by setting aside one wing or ward and assigning dying patients to stay there. A nursing home is not a hospice, and cannot become one by putting out a new sign carrying that name. A hospice must grow from within, is a professional service based on a set of convictions about the nature of life and the meaning of death that make themselves visible in every aspect, however humble or however sophisticated, of hospice work. The visibility of the hospice, in fact, is an important part of it, and one of the identifying marks of a good hospice is that it functions as a smaller community, open at all times to the larger one in which it is understood and welcomed.

Finally, a hospice is a community in need of a home, if it does not already have one. English hospices have usually begun their work in an inpatient facility, and have then reached out to the surrounding neighborhood with domiciliary care services. In America thus far, the situation has been very different. The majority of hospices now springing up consist of interdisciplinary teams committed to caring for people at home, and some include visits to nursing homes, hospitals, or wherever the patient may be at the time. Experience has shown by now, however, that problems under such circumstances often arise which can only be solved in a facility designed or remodeled on hospice principles.

The hospice inpatient unit must function, not as a fortress removed from the rest of society, but as a house of life, a place where dying is seen as a natural part of our human pilgrimage, and where death receives consecration and celebration appropriate to this view. It must offer true welcome, not only to the patient but to his family and friends, to young children, to beloved pets, personal possessions, and whatever amenities belong to the life style of the person who is dying, whether this be food of a certain ethnic variety, or wine and music, or silence and privacy. Provision should be made for the comfort of visitors, including those who, under special circumstances, may wish to stay overnight; and couples should have the opportunity to share physical intimacy even during the final hours, if they wish to do so. Growing plants and garden areas are an important part of the hospice unit, reminders as they are, like music and the other arts, of the forces of renewal in nature and in the human spirit. Medical care must be comprehensive in its dedication to the patient's comfort at all times, and in its attention to any sign that aggressive treatment of the disease might now be appropriate in other surroundings; but the mechanisms for heroic resuscitation and artificial maintenance of life functions do not belong in a hospice inpatient unit. Nursing care here must be maintained at a far higher nurse-patient ratio than is found in hospitals and nursing homes. Members of the clergy must be visibly present and available to those who wish their help at this time, which Elisabeth Kübler-Ross has so well named "the final stage of growth." Trained volunteers are also an extremely important part of the hospice inpatient unit, for they can take on many of the simple, human tasks that are so meaningful in the situation, freeing more highly skilled professionals for other duties. The life of the larger community must flow in and out, quite naturally, here. With constant efforts and vigilance on the part of volunteers and kitchen and janitorial staff, as well as doctors and nurses, this can happen (as it does at St. Christopher's) in an atmosphere of healthful and refreshing cleanliness without the life-denying sterility of the general hospital, and without the rank unpleasant-ness found in all too many of our modern "nursing" and "convalescent" homes.

Inpatient care for hospice patients, when and if it becomes necessary, may have some subtle advantages over the best of the care that can be provided in patients' homes. Families visiting there come into contact with others who are experiencing similar emotions, and help to support one another during the process of loss and bereavement. Many take pleasure in offering small comforts and companionship to dying members of one anothers' families. Patients themselves, brought together at this time, are often able to experience the sort of friendship which is unmasked and thus, however brief, very real and deeply satisfying. "Time," as Dr. Cicely Saunders once remarked, "is not a question of length, it's a question of depth, isn't it?" Witnessing the peaceful sort of death that is made possible by good hospice care, patients and families alike can come to the realization that dying itself is not a horror, and is nothing to be feared, however grievous it may be in terms of parting and, to the bereaved, of loss. A kind of healing can take place and very often does, in hospice patients who have been judged incurable by purely physical standards. Surrounded by love and tenderness, given cleanliness and surcease from bodily pain, they are like travelers who have come briefly to stay in the protected space of an island, there to gather their powers and to free their minds and spirits for the journey into mystery that lies beyond.

Making Circles

CHAPTER 11

We have built ourselves a fortress of personality, and have
thought of ourselves as only a body which we feed, pamper
and display with all our energy. When the body is spoiled
and the fortress crumbles, we are compelled to search for
something more permanent than either.

Getting to Know Saint Joseph's Hospice.

He drew a circle and shut us out
But Love and I found a way to win:
We drew a circle and brought him in.

Barbara Hill (after Edwin Markham)

How many people we all know are like fortresses, guarded and
defended so that it is possible to live beside them day by day, year
by year, catching only a brief, rare glimpse from time to time of
the hidden soul inside. To those who dwell within them, these
fortresses of personality—buttressed by wealth or beauty, wit,
strength, charm, social position, or political power—are often
prisons of a particularly cruel sort. Pride shuts the gates, fear bars
them, and in the sunless, airless space within, nothing can grow.
The process of "failing" and the knowledge that death is drawing
near can be, under such circumstances, a gentle gift, like the
mossy crumbling of old castle walls in lands where peace has
come to stay.

To a certain extent, every one of us is like this. We all develop
defenses in the mere process of living; but if we can learn to
accept our dying as a natural part of the unique and personal

journey of our existence, then the awareness of approaching death can come to us as a release, not from living, but from the merciless demands of ego toward a richer life, a way of being which is filled with the freedom children have to wonder and to dream, to marvel, to experience each event in time and space as limitless, mysterious, unique. It is the loved and wanted child who claims this gift of spiritual wisdom as his birthright, and who never quite relinquishes it, however harsh his fate may be in later years.

To be wanted in such a way, circled round not with moats and walls but with meadow spaces of love and freedom, is the deathright of each individual who has become once again in terminal illness like a child, helpless, undefended, incompetent, and useless by worldly standards, and thus fully qualified at last for reentry into the Kingdom of Heaven. The caring circle of the hospice community responds as a matter of principle and conviction to this view of human value—a view which is not new, but radical in the sense of being rooted deeply in traditional sources of familial and communal vitality.

The making of these vital circles is a task being undertaken by teams gathering faster in the United States today than any book could be written about them. Newsletters, brochures, articles, and notices of forums and seminars on hospice development now clutter the files of those who have expressed interest in the subject, and a rare, heartening sort of collection it is. Words leap from these pages that refresh the soul and lend new dimension to all our present thinking on the subject of medical responsibility. Here we are not assaulted by robotlike statements about "total package costs," "credibility gaps," or "function-utilizations" and we do not hear the leer of the adman promising "projects with real payoff." The message, instead, from a rapidly growing hospice group in the Southeast is: "only spirit-filled doctors, nurses and clergy can determine the new medical thought and practice necessary for such a radical departure from the pragmatic into the wholistic approach." And, from a small farming town in California, "the purpose of this newsletter is to introduce you, our living community, to Mercy Hospice. We declare ourselves as joining hands and hearts with others in the hospice movement throughout the world, that have come before us and who will follow. We have been awakened to the need. We dedicate ourselves to the solution and we ask for your support. . . ."

"The hospice movement," said Elisabeth Kübler-Ross in California on January 27, 1977, "is the finest organization for change in this country today."

American hospices are appearing now in many different forms, with the models provided by St. Christopher's and other outstanding English hospices, and by the work of Dr. Kübler-Ross translated and transmuted by the necessities of differing situations. In the past two months (as these words are being written) some 20 more new hospice groups have joined the 50 noted in April, 1977, on the map at New Haven's Hospice, Inc. In the state of California alone, 22 teams are now organizing or already at work. Few of the new hospice teams are prepared as yet to begin treating patients; most are in the process of seeking community support, and struggling with the usual problems of funding, staffing, and interior organization. Nearly all are being founded by physicians and nurses who plan to begin by offering skilled home care to the terminally ill, hoping to have inpatient units of their own in time. The movement is one, essentially, of professional people in the health-care fields who find the present situation intolerable, who discover support for their view among members of the clergy and enlightened laypeople, and who are willing to devote enormous amounts of time, energy, and personal sacrifice to the cause of providing better and more appropriate care in the future, to the terminally ill.

There is a tension at present within the movement itself between those who believe that true hospice care can be provided within the environs of the general hospital, and those who believe that a separate, fully autonomous inpatient unit is necessary. As President Carter has pointed out, one of the reasons for high-cost hospital care at present is that the patient who is admitted must pay at the same time for the beds in the hospital which are empty, and it might seem a simple solution to administrators simply to put "hospice patients" into those empty beds in order to balance the budget. However, the experience of St. Christopher's, of New Haven's Hospice, Inc., and of Hospice of Marin serves to suggest that a separate unit is necessary; and a study of several other hospice models now operating in North America and Great Britain tends further to confirm this view. The "caring community" is a process of human interaction so foreign.to the function assumed over the years by our general hospitals, and its practical needs are so unlike those of the acute-care system that it cannot do its work without autonomy. The few in-hospital units that can honestly be called hospices are the work of remarkably determined individuals who struggle daily against the system around them, and who find themselves too often in a position of unsatisfactory compromise.

One of the finest of the in-hospital efforts is to be found at St. Luke's Hospital Center, beside the magnificent Cathedral of St. John The Divine, on the upper west side of Manhattan, New York City. Here at St. Luke's, spiritual care of the ill has long been traditional, along with the practice of scientific medicine, teaching, and research. A team has recently been formed among staff members here, calling itself a Hospice Pilot Project and in April of 1975 began offering special services to terminally ill patients and their families. Pain and symptom control are managed with the aid of hospice medications and patients on this service, while they are not placed separately from others, are given special opportunities to have visitors, to ask and receive help with family problems, and to discuss their condition with trained counselors if they wish to do so. Many of these patients are enabled to return to their homes, given supportive help by members of the hospice team, and every effort is made, whether they are in the hospital or at home, to help them live as fully as possible until death comes. Follow-up bereavement counseling is also offered by the team, which consists of a nurse-coordinator, a chaplain, a physician specializing in oncology, two nurses, a social worker, three part-time psychiatrists and four volunteers.

One of the aims of the St. Luke's Pilot Project, says Chaplain David Pyle, has been to share the knowledge of modern hospice care with the rest of the hospital community simply by giving them the opportunity to see it in action. The present arrangement has the advantage on that score of allowing the hospice team to work in many different units; and the sight of a terminally ill patient comfortable and alert, given full human rights and privileges in the situation, obviously serves as a powerful witness to the hospice philosophy. Yet the visitor feels (and the patients themselves must be acutely aware) that on every side are differently directed disciplines with all the machinery, the drama, and the haste and dispatch of acute-care medicine. Patients and their families here are still trapped too in the insurance reimbursement system which is geared to expensive, aggressive treatment of disease. A separate unit is obviously needed so that the circle of this hospice community may in time be visibly drawn and recognized financially, as well as medically and socially, in appropriate ways. In a separate unit, friends and families could gather freely, life on hospital grounds could proceed until its ending on a far more normal basis, and medical care of the patient could continue at the same time in the hospice way, which is intensive in the personal, rather than the technological sense. The program of St. Luke's is impressive now in its expertise and in its lovingkindness. No doubt, many hospitals in the United States will undergo some gentle changes in the direction of *hospitality* as the result of efforts such as this, for here the yeast is definitely in the loaf; but the situation as a whole indicates that better provision must be made in the future for patients, families—and for staff—who are actively involved in the hospice process of terminal care.

Halfway across the country, in downtown Saint Paul, Minnesota, another hospice model is now in operation, struggling to become a community within hospital walls. Here at Bethesda Lutheran Hospital physicians fight disease, and teaching and research have their place as well; but in conversation with Robert S. Brown, M.D., of the new Hospice Unit, we hear the word "healing" at least as often as we hear the word "cure." The wholeness of the patient as an individual is the primary concern of this remarkably sensitive and articulate young oncologist who, together with his colleagues, Dr. Richard E. YaDeau and Dr. Donald L. Foss, has brought hospice principles to the care of terminally ill cancer patients at Bethesda Lutheran. Here in a separate unit within the hospital, patients undergoing active treatment of disease are received together with those who cannot be cured and whose care is technically palliative. In either case, the person is perceived as a being involved in the "spiritual continuum" which Dr. Brown and his associates see as the heart of the hospice process.

Patients and their families are met on arrival here with an immediate opportunity to discuss at length with staff, not only their physical condition, but their personal feelings on any subject of importance to them. Psychological and spiritual problems are considered from the first to be as significant as the presence of physical disease, and the family is recognized as an important part of the healing process. The patient's pastor, if he has one or requests one, is given full access to medical charts and takes part in the treatment plan—an idea so sensible that it is surprising to think how very seldom such a thing happens within our hospitals today. Here, the pastor is welcomed as a professional equal in the structure of the care-giving team.

Dr. Brown has devised a series of diagrams which he is fond of using in the process of explaining the philosophical basis of his work. Here again we find the image of a circle, indicating in this case the wholeness of what he calls the "triune being" of man. Three overlapping arcs within this circle delineate physical, psychological and spiritual components of the individual, equal in size and interlocking in function. The *cure* of cancer, Dr. Brown says, means restoration of the integrity of a single part only—the physical—and *healing* is seen as the ultimate aim whether or not curing is possible. To heal is to enable the patient to achieve integration, to realize himself, whatever his physical condition, as a whole person. When the physical component cannot be restored, then the spiritual and psychological elements begin to assume greater importance, and the staff of this hospice unit are prepared to respond to that.

For control of pain the Bethesda unit uses a basic program

developed in Seattle, combining methadone with other medications designed to relieve anxiety and depression, and administered
in the hospice fashion regularly, round the clock, rather than PRN
(as needed). Activities and visitors in the 20-bed ward are a
constant aid, as well, in maintaining the patient's comfort and
sense of participation in the ongoing processes of life. "We
believe in the importance of touching," says Dr. Brown, "of hands
reaching out, giving and receiving." Hands touch here, and they
also participate in prayer. The Monday morning staff meetings
were at first ordinary discussion periods and support sessions, but
during the past year since the founding of the unit, it has come to
seem natural for this group to pray together as well. Hard
medicine and what one pastor likes to call "solid spirituality" are
combined here, as at St. Christopher's. Side by side with expert
surgery, chemotherapy, and all other modern techniques for the
medical control of cancer, at Bethesda Hospice there is a practice
(on occasion, for patients who wish it) of prayer with laying-on-of-
hands. The aim of a hospice, Dr. Cicely Saunders once said, is
"supported reality." Here is a team obviously willing and able to
support all parts of the suffering person's existence, not excluding
those which are ineluctably mysterious. Death, when it comes, is
consecrated here, but in the meantime, life is enriched in every
way possible and fully celebrated. With the aid of a small grant
recently received, the unit is now organizing a coordinated home-
care program, and support groups for staff members and families
are also being formed. In time, the full range of hospice services
will undoubtedly be developed here as well as such a program can
hope to be, within the fortress walls of the American hospital
system.

The operational balance, however, in any unit such as this is a
matter of great delicacy. The problem of appropriate insurance
coverage for palliative care still looms, and may continue to do so
as far as American hospice teams are concerned until present
reimbursement systems are sensibly amended. There are cancer
patients in active treatment who need, for their own protection,
to be isolated at times from the life of a hospice community; and a
hospital ward, however pleasantly equipped, cannot offer the

homelike atmosphere of a physically independent unit. The work of Dr. Brown and his colleagues at Bethesda Lutheran, under such circumstances, is a truly inspired *tour de force;* and it is to be hoped that it is a harbinger of change throughout our present system as well.

North of the Canadian border at the Royal Victoria Hospital in Montreal is a well-established Palliative Care Service (PCS) whose operational problems have been eased, not only by the support of the hospital, the Ministère des Affaires Sociales, and private philanthropy, but by the acceptance of this mode of care for the terminally ill by the National Health Service of Canada. Under the direction of Dr. Balfour M. Mount, Associate Professor of Surgery (Urology) at McGill University and head of the PCS, a separate unit has been set up within the hospital, where patients in the terminal stages of malignant disease are given medical, psychological, and spiritual support on hospice principles. Staff leaders, trained at St. Christopher's and instructed by the teachings of Dr. Elisabeth Kübler-Ross, make every effort to improve the quality of life remaining for those who cannot be cured, firmly believing (and demonstrating in their daily work) that there is never a situation in terminal illness in which "nothing more can be done." Pain and symptom control here are managed on a round-the-clock basis with careful titration to match the changing needs of the individual patient; for acute pain, the Hospice Mix here combines oral narcotic agents (methadone and others have been used as well as morphine) with a phenothiazine and a variety of other medications. Other forms of discomfort and dysfunction are met with a great variety of pharmacological and physical therapies, and by devoted nursing care by a small but intensely concerned and attentive staff of medical professionals and volunteers.

It is a cheerful, small unit here at the Royal Victoria, somewhat reminiscent of St. Christopher's in miniature, with brightly colored coverlets on all the beds, curtains and plants, reclining chairs for patients who are more comfortable in them than in their beds, and personal belongings of patients much in evidence.

Visitors mingle freely with patients in an atmosphere of friendly, and at times frankly emotional give-and-take. Family members are encouraged to help with patient care, to bring in special foods that might give pleasure, and to develop relationships with one another as well as supportive habits of practical and emotional assistance with other patients. Montreal is a city, like many in the United States, of great variety in cultural backgrounds. Some 40 percent of citizens here are French Canadian (mostly Roman Catholic), 40 percent English of various denominations, and the other 20 percent from backgrounds as widely differing as Greek and Chinese. In the hospital unit, as well as in the coordinated home-care service, staff members must be prepared to deal with the expectations of people whose standards are as different as their various backgrounds; staff themselves differ widely, and this has obviously presented some special problems in the formation of community. The admirable 516-page *Report of the Palliative Care Service (Rapport de la Service des Soins Palliatifs)*, published in 1976 with French on one page, English on another, gives evidence of exhaustive research and continuous evaluation of the project, and is filled with medical and sociological data of every appropriate sort, but is at the same time a reminder of the cultural dichotomies in the situation.

Members of staff here are frank to admit that it has been a difficult challenge to sort out their religious and philosophical attitudes about dealing with death. Those who had no personal systems developed felt particularly uncomfortable at first, working with others who held firm, though often differing points of view. The decision, made early in the establishment of the Service, to keep members of this staff working together rather than transferring them back and forth from the main body of the hospital has obviously been a helpful one. With great patience and a determination to maintain open communications on subjects of ultimate value, the hospice staff has drawn closer together in time; social events in particular are greatly enjoyed by the group; and the notable success of the Service as a professional venture has tended to heighten morale. The denial of death, and the comparative neglect (or inappropriate overtreatment) of dying patients has been a problem as severe in the Canadian medical system as in America; and Dr. Mount and his staff now have firm evidence in their two-year Pilot Project that hospice methods are better medically and morally, as well as being less costly than previous methods of management.

In many ways this Palliative Care Service, with its inpatient unit, its home-care team, consultation and follow-up bereavement group, manages well to duplicate the work of a hospice such as St. Christopher's within the general hospital setting. Much here is missing, however: the space, the children, the elderly residents gathering informally with staff, young people, students, volunteers, and visitors, as well as patients in the ordinary course of events, and above all, perhaps, the sense of being in a place where many nonmedical things are happening simply because they are neighborly and interesting. It is difficult indeed for living and dying to be mixed in together well and naturally, as hospice people believe they ought to be, unless there is some real distance—particularly psychological distance, of course—between the hospice itself and the hospital. The economic realities may force a good deal of compromise on issues such as this in America today, but it is always possible to keep working, even so, toward the eventual ideal.

Physically separate, yet connected, and yet autonomous: a paradox, it may seem; but there is a fine model for this sort of hospice available in England today. On the grounds of Churchill Hospital in the university town of Oxford, a modest but very attractive small building has recently been constructed called Sir Michael Sobell House, and also referred to as the Continuing Care Unit of the hospital itself. Like most hospices in America and in England, this unit has depended on a combination of public and private funding sources for its creation: a gift from Sir Michael Sobell (President of the National Society for Cancer Relief), foundations and utilities supplied by the National Health Service (NHS), and local appeals to complete and to furnish the building. Although Sir Michael Sobell House is now technically part of the NHS, it operates with professional autonomy under the direction of Dr. R. G. Twycross, who for a number of years was chief of Clinical Pharmacology at St. Christopher's.

Though the hospital itself looms nearby (and will soon be physically connected by a covered corridor) this free-standing unit looks rather like a pleasant country house of brick and glass, with its own gardens around it and an atmosphere entirely of its own. Patients' rooms and wards are airy and open to the outside, and natural wood has been used freely throughout the interior, so that the feeling of it is not at all dreary or institutional. Twenty-five patients can be accommodated in four wards of five beds each and five single rooms; there is also a separate kitchen, a laundry and cleaner, a hairdressing facility, a treatment room, and offices and a seminar room for staff. A spacious day room has magazines, plants, and television for patients and visitors, adjacent to a quiet room chapel and reception area. Two important innovations in hospice design were noted here: one, that round tables are provided in the wards so that patients can share companionable mealtimes together, and also that two "bed-sitter" rooms, sharing a private bath, are an integral part of the unit for the use of visiting relatives. Patients who are able to be up and about mix easily here with members of staff and visitors, including children, who are especially welcomed with various decorations and treats designed to delight them. The character of this small community on hospital grounds is maintained, in these various ways, as a cozy and homelike way station for patients and their families in times of special need. Everything about the unit suggests medical expertise, yet nothing here is strange, forbidding, or frightening.

The character of the Medical Director is, as usual, an important element in this hospice situation. For many years pain control has been, one might almost say, the passion of Dr. Robert Twycross. Although he is an immensely precise and cautious statistician who has published quantities of charts and studies on the use of modern drugs, and who continues to collect data constantly on his daily rounds, he is also tuned, in a very sensitive way, to the personal qualities of each individual patient, and to the complexity of pain which is psychological and spiritual as well as physical. With a modest apology that "I hope this does not sound too pious," Dr. Twycross has drawn up a list of Ten Commandments for physicians dealing with the pain of cancer:

1. Thou Shalt not Assume that the Patient's Pain is due to the Malignant Process.
2. Thou Shalt try Simple Analgesics in the First Instance.
3. Thou Shalt not be Afraid of Narcotic Drugs.
4. Thou Shalt not Prescribe Inadequate Amounts of any Analgesic.
5. Thou Shalt not Use the Abbreviation PRN.
6. Thou Shalt Take into Consideration the Patient's Feelings.
7. Thou Shalt Provide Support for the Whole Family.
8. Thou Shalt not Limit thy Approach Simply to the use of Drugs.
9. Thou Shalt not be Afraid to ask Colleague's Advice.
10. Thou Shalt have an air of Quiet Confidence and Cautious Optimism.

Together with Dr. Saunders and other experts in the field, Dr. Twycross has made the extensive studies which now allow very severe pain to be controlled to a remarkable degree, while maintaining alertness of patients in modern hospices. By means of polypharmacy—the use of many different medications in a single situation—he adjusts each patient's regimen, and readjusts it as often as necessary to keep the individual comfortable and in a normal frame of mind while outmaneuvering the central nervous system's messages of agony. Bone pain, for example, which is apt to be particularly savage and intractable, is managed under the system with the aid of powerful anti-inflammatory drugs, as well as the usual Hospice Mix containing diamorphine as its basic ingredient. The "double nature" of pain is carefully monitored, met not only with proper analgesics and tender care for the individual, but with an honest relationship which the patient can trust. Dr. Twycross does not believe in concealing the fact that they are dying from terminal patients. However, he would not press such information on them, any more than he would press upon them his own (Christian) religious views. If patients indicate, sometimes in rather subtle ways, that they wish to face facts in an open discussion, then staff members here are alert to that. "Patients always appreciate gentle truth," Dr. Twycross says. His stance of cautious optimism is designed, not to fool the patient for whom there is no reasonable hope of cure, but in recognition of the fact that reason is not always correct in any case; and in order to reassure the patient that the days ahead, whatever happens, will not be filled with humiliation and physical torment. These attitudes in themselves are undoubtedly an important element in the success of his pain-control program, and in the success of the many hospice directors here and abroad who have used his research as the launching point for their own methodologies.

The advantages of such a unit, attached to a great hospital center, yet separate and autonomous in its procedure, are obviously considerable. Dr. Twycross works closely with colleagues at Churchill, counsels conveniently with them on matters involving patients within the hospital itself, and can readily return his own patients for aggressive treatment such as radiation therapy, in cases where he believes it might be helpful. There are economic advantages in that all expenses do not have to be met separately by the hospice unit; and the reputation of Churchill Hospital is undoubtedly reassuring to many patients and families who come here. However, in its placement some distance away from the mainstream of life in Oxford town, and in its connection with the hospital rather than the community at large, Sir Michael Sobell House must take extra care not to be overwhelmed by the institutional atmosphere at hand. Vigilance of this sort may turn out to be even more necessary in American hospital-hospices than it is in England because essentially the issue is one of authority. When a patient goes to Sir Michael Sobell House, Dr. Twycross is in charge. There is no question about it, and Dr. Twycross does not have to waste time and energy negotiating for control over his own procedures. While Americans tend to imagine that our own institutions are more democratic than this, and while we talk a great deal about "team decision-making," the fact is that insurance companies, lawyers, and bureaucrats have taken control over all too many of our own medical procedures; so that in actual practice, we have only managed to substitute outside authorities for those within. Meantime we have allowed people who are not medical professionals to build little empires for themselves all around the edges of the situation, and it is the amenities of these entrepreneurs that we pay for when we are sick.

Humble beginnings, it seems clear by now, are one of the important hallmarks of the hospice movement. Careful research, thorough training, the seeking of funds from many sources, and the gradual development of a sense of community-within-community are the necessary prerequisites for the growth of this very new, yet very old form of *hospitality*. When the hospice begins, as most in the United States are now beginning, independently in the sense of being without any direct hospital connection or support, some problems are multiplied but others are avoided altogether. Both here and in England, models are now available for this method of procedure; and although Orlando, Florida, is a long way from the town of Worthing in Sussex, England, we can find similar patterns of development, studying the progress of independent hospices in both places. The establishment of St. Barnabas' Home in Sussex was a seven-year community effort, led by a physician who had studied the pioneering work of Dr. Saunders in the course of caring for his own cancer patients. Hospice Orlando, incorporated only this year (April, 1977) is now beginning its long struggle under the direction of a medical oncologist, Dr. Daniel C. Hadlock, whose principles are also those of Dr. Saunders and St. Christopher's.

In many ways, Orlando is a typical American community—a small town grown into a moderately large city with its cluster of suburban towns around it—and like the town of Worthing, it is pleasantly green, unassumingly handsome, and filled with great numbers of those extraordinary people who are usually known as "average citizens." There is no special reason why, in either of these communities, the needs of the terminally ill should have become a compelling subject of research and public attention and yet, because the problem is a universal one, and because of the presence here of people willing to work with it, both Worthing and Orlando now have hospices.

"A Very Special Way of Caring" is the way Hospice Orlando people describe their services. It is a small group: three physicians, a clergyman, and a handful of concerned laypeople are on the board. Of the volunteer staff of ten now actively on the job, providing hospice home care to patients in the area, half are trained RNs or LPNs donating their time. The hospice office is in the home of Dr. and Mrs. Hadlock at the moment, and with the help of Joyce Yager, who serves as secretary and administrative assistant, plus message-answering services, staff are available on a 24-hour-a-day, 7-days-a-week basis. In the past six months of 1977 63 terminally ill patients and their families have been given hospice care; and all of this has been accomplished with the aid of only one small grant (a City Service Award) and one paid staff member. Like Hospice of Marin (and like St. Barnabas' in England as well) this has been a grassroots operation, the work of medical professionals, clergy, and members of the community who gathered gradually around the physician who offered leadership in the situation.

Lacking an inpatient unit at present, Dr. Hadlock's immediate aim is to keep patients comfortably at home during the last stages of their illness, providing that this is what they want and that it seems best for the family, too. Each case is monitored carefully from day to day, with attention to the psychological and spiritual needs of the family unit, as well as the medical and the practical. Nursing techniques are modeled on the practices of St. Christopher's, and a Hospice Mix is given for pain similar to those used at Hospice, Inc. and Hospice of Marin, consisting usually of morphine with Compazine in water or cherry syrup. Consent and cooperation of the patient's own physician is necessary, and there must be a "primary care person" in the home who is willing to assist and cooperate with the hospice program. Close relations are maintained with consultants in radiation oncology and other disciplines of aggressive treatment, throughout; at present, only patients with a diagnosis of terminal cancer can be admitted to the program, though it is hoped that other incurably ill people may be helped by Hospice Orlando in time.

Bereavement is considered a medical problem by this team, and their program includes support of family members as long as needed. Many in the hospice are devout Christians who find prayer an important part of their regular staff meetings, but their aim in the community is "to support every patient and family dealing with the distress caused by incurable disease without bias. Then they can have true freedom to develop the ability to deal with their situation according to their own understanding."

In the modern world there has lately sprung up an interesting new science, or craft, perhaps, known to the initiate as "grantsmanship." Experts in this field organize and reorganize vast quantities of printed material and produce documents designed, with enormous enthusiasm and skill, to empty as painlessly as possible the pockets of all who behold them. Doubtless this is a worthy profession, but it must be admitted that no member of it, however eager or astute, could invent a plea more eloquent than the simple statement of Hospice Orlando that it seeks funds from those "who support our goals and who some day may have need of our services." It is one thing to write a check, pleasantly benevolent and delightfully tax-deductible, for an individual, a group, or an institution removed at safe distance from the realities of one's own existence. It is quite another to make an investment in a project promising decency of treatment for one's own kin and neighbors and even, perhaps, for oneself. As soon as actual patient care began late in 1976, public support of Hospice Orlando began rapidly to increase; newspapers took note of the extraordinary relief from pain and anguish offered by its system, and donations began coming in from grateful friends and family members of those who had received hospice support. Eventually, the team plans to bill patients for that part of their care which is covered by insurance or other third-party reimbursement agencies, and the balance of cost will be covered, as it is now, by donation. If Hospice Orlando is to survive, and if it is to continue to grow so as to serve the entire community, grants and donations must be generous.

"Where will we find the money?" This was the question asked only a few years ago in Sussex by Dr. F. R. Gusterson, director of the small, independent hospice known as St. Barnabas' Home. To this, a clergyman friend of his replied, "This work is vitally necessary, isn't it? Then if you all do your part well, it will succeed." Faith, in the hospice movement, is not merely a matter of thinking fine thoughts, but of recognizing practical realities, and responding to them. The people of Worthing were aware that better methods of care were needed for the dying, in particular for those suffering in the final stages of cancer. When Dr. Gusterson was heard explaining the hospice concept, community interest began to gather around him, rather gradually at first, but as the news spread, with increasing intensity. The immediate aim of this group was an inpatient unit, purpose-built, to supplement the enlightened home care which was already being given by Dr. Gusterson to many patients in the area. Very early it was decided that professional fund-raisers would not be hired. Founders felt that the hospice must have its roots firmly planted within the community; and a series of determined efforts during the 1960s brought response to pleas for funds and help of various kinds, from people in many professions, many different churches and different walks of life. Charitable trusts offered donations and interest-free loans, and a gift of £10,000 was received from the National Society for Cancer Relief, while small amounts continued to arrive in a slow but steady stream from concerned local citizens. Dr. Cicely Saunders lent support with a moving address before a large audience of townspeople, giving them further evidence of the nature and the value of hospice work. Finally, on December 7, 1971, ground was broken for the hospice in a fine ceremony during which the Mayor of Worthing drove a bulldozer onto the site.

It is a charming building now, very simply and inexpensively constructed with prefabricated units set in the shape of a cross at the end of a curving drive. Large areas of glass face patio and garden. There are 30 patient beds, six in single rooms, the others in small bays of four beds each in larger wards. The central lounge for patients and visitors serves also, when curtains are drawn from the recessed altar, as a chapel for weekly, interdenominational services. Registered as a charity, St. Barnabas' welcomes all who are in need of its care. Dr. Gusterson, the Director, known here informally as "Dr. Gus," is a devoutly religious person with a twinkle in his eye, who believes that the work of a hospice is in itself a form of worship, and of prayer. However, "we all feel very strongly," he says, "that the religious side of our work must be played in very low key. Our main concern is to give patients love and care; where we get the strength to do this is our own affair. Any member of staff is always willing to discuss spiritual matters with a patient, but all feel that the patient must first indicate a wish to do so. The general atmosphere of St. Barnabas' is one of 'prayer in action.' "

Patients (some long-term, most in the final stages of cancer) are kept comfortable with medical and nursing techniques modeled on St. Christopher's, and Dr. Gusterson has taught general practitioners in the area how to prescribe for patients remaining at home. A well-trained Domiciliary Care team now operates within a radius of about seven miles, including in their attention all aspects of the patient's life, from a family disagreement to a chimney that is leaking. "Don't just treat the pain," says Dr. Gusterson, "treat the situation." A chimney leaking during a Sussex winter is something to be taken seriously indeed; like some of the nonsensical discomforts provided by our modern hospitals, such a thing shouldn't happen to a person who is sick.

Within the hospice (which *is* a hospice, because of what it does, although it is called St. Barnabas' Home) the situation is pleasant, the mood is somehow at the same time both tranquil and lively, and the food is extraordinarily good. Patients who are at all able to enjoy eating look forward to mealtimes, which together with a constant round of extra teas and treats, have caused visitors to complain, after a day or two, of bulging waistlines. Many members of the nursing staff work here part time, bringing with them fresh bits of news from the larger community. Family members, friends, and volunteers are very much in evidence also, so that there is no sense of being isolated or "put away" for the people here who are ill. A favorite daily ritual for everyone is the feeding of the birds that come to visit regularly, and this touching ceremony has been memorialized in a prayer written by an eight-year-old visitor: "Dear Jesus, please bless and help all the Doctors, Nurses and ill people belonging to St. Barnabas' Home; make them better and please let the birds sing outside their windows. Amen."

The key word here is "belonging." Medical professionals, helpers, patients, and visitors here all belong to one another and to the hospice which is so obviously an important and an honored part of the larger community. This is a satisfaction nearly as difficult for physicians and nurses to find in the ordinary hospital today as it is for the terminally ill. It is a kind of death, whether one is giving or receiving medical care, to find one's humanity measured out by the computer, divided into layers by a system designed along lines of military efficiency, and controlled by the functional demands of corporate machinery. The hospice mode will prove a tremendous boon to medical people who have suffered a sense of personal injury in this sort of situation. The need to be needed is a powerful human trait. It is, actually, one of the main reasons why many people enter the medical professions, only to be frustrated by the impersonality of the present systems. Hospice work demands special training, it is hard work and there is grief in it. Nevertheless, it offers benefits far beyond price, to individuals who are suited by nature to this sort of endeavor. A hospice nurse in California remarked recently, "I did two tours of duty in Vietnam in a MASH unit, and the work I have been doing here lately, believe me, is harder. But for the effort I put into it, the personal rewards are so tremendous that I can't begin to describe them."

Sometimes we forget that the word "professional" once

referred, by definition, not to the attainment of superior technical skills, but to the profession of a faith. In the hospice movement the ancient meaning of the word is now recovered, and, combined with newer uses of it, emerges greatly refreshed. The offer of healing where cure is impossible, the donation of time and energy without guarantee of material reward, and the launching of new modes of caring into the chaos of a hostile, nervous, and fragmented society: all are acts of profession, and of faith that there is real meaning and solid value in human life. In the service of this central profession of belief, hospice people bring to bear the skills that have been more recently considered professional: medicine, nursing, architectural design, psychiatric and pastoral counseling, art, social work, administration and communication, fund-raising and engineering, teaching and research. For that matter, the cook in the hospice kitchen and the janitor who washes the windows here is as much of a professional as the oncologist or the pharmacologist, for all members of the hospice community depend on one another's commitment to the value of the work.

For this reason, it is not surprising to find so many religious people deeply involved in the movement today. The medieval tradition of honoring the dying, and of offering them especially devoted and attentive care, has never entirely vanished from American society as long as there have been groups at work such as the Sisters of the House of Calvary in New York City, and spiritually dedicated individuals like Rose Hawthorne Lathrop (Nathaniel Hawthorne's daughter), willing and able to establish Homes with decent standards of care for the terminally ill. Long before the modern aspects of the movement began to emerge, these religious professionals were offering refuge and tender care to incurable patients who would otherwise have been very badly treated by the rest of society, and their example should not be forgotten in our present efforts to develop medical and administrative aspects of hospice care. One of the most interesting modern hospice models, in fact, is an ancient nursing home founded by a religious order, which has kept these elements of its character intact while managing at the same time to transform itself into a first-rate, modern medical facility.

In the heart of London's East End, a district rich in history and cultural flavor, though economically quite poor, the Irish Sisters of Charity have been welcoming terminally ill patients (and some long-term patients as well) at St. Joseph's Hospice for the past 72 years. It was here that Dr. Cicely Saunders did some of her important pioneering work in pain control before opening St. Christopher's; and like St. Christopher's Hospice, this 100-bed facility now combines the most advanced of therapeutic, medical techniques with the conviction that patients and their families must be offered a nourishing ground of spiritual and emotional support.

Set among busy streets, the main building of St. Joseph's is a three-story structure of brick with glass walls and balconies opening to a protected garden-patio area. Patients are received in modest and somewhat spare but cheerful four- and six-bedded wards, each with its own color scheme and floral-printed bedspreads. Around each bed are curtains which can be drawn for privacy; each patient has a locker for personal belongings, and flowers are on every bedside table. On each floor is a pleasantly furnished day-room, where patients who are able to be up and about generally spend their mornings visiting together. Most people here are elderly, and suffering from terminal cancer; only 10 percent stay longer than three weeks; but long-term patients are carefully mixed in among the dying in an effort to maintain a sense of continuity and community in the wards. The aim of the hospice staff is to encourage earlier referrals from the neighborhood, so that patients can be here for a period of one or two months.

The rhythm of daily life at St. Joseph's (though members of any group or faith are entirely welcome) is that of a strongly liturgical religious order. Chapel bells ring three times a day, and all work in the hospice ceases for a moment of prayer. Dr. Richard Lamerton, director of the Domiciliary Care Service, who is himself a Quaker, holds daily staff conferences which begin with a scripture reading, and members of this team meet after luncheon each day for a quiet period of half an hour or more designed to replenish their sense of inner serenity, by means of silent contemplation or the practice of such meditative arts as needle-point and calligraphy.

The relief of pain is seen at St. Joseph's Hospice as a religious duty and a "most marvellous act of mercy." Diamorphine (heroin) is given regularly—not PRN—in an oral mix sometimes combined with cocaine and gin, or, when necessary, injected intra-muscularly or subcutaneously in amounts as large as necessary to prevent pain and to bring relaxation into a maximal balance with alertness. Antiemetics, steroids, phenothiazines, and other pallia-tive medications are used, where indicated, as well. Careful attention is given to personal hygiene and to medical and emotional difficulties associated with terminal illness: embarrass-ment over incontinence, for example, being considered as signif-icant a problem to work with as the practical issues presented by the condition. Physicians and nurses at St. Joseph's have found (as have staff at other authentic hospices) that drug addiction is not a problem. Very rarely do any signs of it occur, and if they do, they can be controlled by shifts in the type of medication or disregarded in the case of a patient who is at the point of death. By offering initial dosages high enough to block the memory of pain and fear of its recurrence, and by treating the patient as a respected individual, staff here are able to bring about relaxation to such a degree that drug use can often be greatly reduced, even as the disease itself progresses; and many patients who have come into the hospice in agony are enabled to return to their homes, remaining comfortably there under the supervision of the Domiciliary Care team.

The issue of mercy-killing is faced forthrightly at St. Joseph's Hospice. "If anyone really wants euthanasia," says Dr. Lamerton, "he must have pretty poor doctors and nurses." And he continues, "It is not that the question of euthanasia is right or wrong, desirable or repugnant, practical or unworkable. It is just that it is irrelevant. We as doctors have a duty so to care for our patients that they never ask to be killed off. If we fail in our duty let us not turn to the politicians asking them to extricate us from the mess."

More than one new hospice team in the United States has discovered that local physicians balk at the news of modern hospice-care methods, fearing most these two issues: drug addiction and euthanasia. A talk with Dr. Lamerton and a visit with the nursing Sisters at St. Joseph's, their patients calm and alert, conversing sensibly and moving about in a perfectly normal manner, might persuade these physicians that their alarm is entirely unnecessary. Euthanasia is wholly contrary to hospice principles, not only because it becomes an irrelevant issue in this mode of care, but because, as Dr. Lamerton says, "Dying is still a part of living. In this period a man may learn some of his life's most important lessons." At St. Luke's in New York, Chaplain David Pyle echoes this view. "A dying man," he says, "came recently under our care, and learned for the first time in his life that it was possible for him to trust another human being." In America, the widely noted research of Dr. Elisabeth Kübler-Ross, and her manner of caring for her own patients, has paved the way for better understanding that this indeed can happen—that dying can be a time of great personal growth, if only the right conditions are offered for it.

Trust of the institution—of any medical institution whatever—is a problem in the neighborhood of St. Joseph's, where fear runs deep of "being put away in 'ospital"; therefore the Domiciliary Care Service has served an unusually crucial need here. In the year 1976, this team cared for 263 patients, 44.9 percent of them dying at home. Relations with the community are helped, too, by the atmosphere created at the regular Thursday clinics for outpatients. Here the ill person comes, not only for care and contact with physicians, but for the sort of outing which is rare in an economically depressed area, including a chance to chat and gossip comfortably with other patients and volunteers over pots of tea and plates of cookies. Nurses already live on the grounds of St. Joseph's, and a new structure is now being added to receive chronically ill young adults: a move which will further broaden and deepen the quality of community life at the hospice, and help to remove from it the stigma of a place where people come only to die.

At Yale University in June of 1976, Dr. Cicely Saunders introduced her remarks on the hospice concept by saying, "I am here from St. Christopher's, which, by the way, is neither a Shangri-La nor a death-house." Her audience, though it was largely composed of professionals in the health care fields, responded with somewhat nervous laughter; and the quality of that laughter represented, I suppose, the difficulty many of us still have in coping with what is real, rather than taking refuge in fantasies of horror or of perfection. The hospice movement, however, is firmly rooted in reality. The facts of human life are its base: physical facts, psychological facts, historical facts, economic facts, and not least of all, the fact that spiritual forces are at work in us constantly, however little we may be aware of them. The hospice process, whatever its location, its staffing and funding problems, or the stage of development reached by a particular facility, is faith in action. Humanists may prefer to call it faith in humanity; atheists may insist that it has nothing to do with God; and many people within the movement itself are willing to work for the comfort of the dying without believing in any sort of afterlife. Nevertheless, faith is the heart of this process and this profession, simply because there is no other force (by whatever name) that could cause people to behave toward one another as they do in the hospice situation. Physical care of those who are "failing" can be bought and paid for. "Useless" members of society can be dealt with by legislation, revolution, or simple elimination. The energy for hospice work, however, must come from an entirely different source.

The fact that, at present, the source appears to be strongly Christian should not distract our attention from the broader implications and possibilities of the movement as a whole. The courtesies of the Orient and the traditional hospitality of Abraham are as much a part of the hospice vision as Christian liturgy. The hospice is a way station designed for the refreshment of all who are on the final journey; and it is the kind of space created here that matters most. As Henri Nouwen writes in *Reaching Out:*

> Indeed, the stranger has to be received in a free and friendly space where he can reveal his gifts and become our friend. ... Really honest receptivity means inviting the stranger into our world on his or her terms, not on ours. When we say, "You can be my guest if you believe what I believe, think the way I think and behave as I do," we offer love under a condition or for a price. This leads easily to exploitation, making hospitality into a business. In our world in which so many religious convictions, ideologies and life styles come into increasing contact with each other, it is more important than ever to realize that it belongs to the essence of a Christian spirituality to receive our fellow human beings into our world without imposing our religious viewpoint, ideology or way of doing things on them as a condition for love, friendship and care.

It is this kind of love, friendship, and care that hospice workers offer, whether their base is a hospital, a haven created by an ancient religious order, or a tiny office in a physician's private home. The personal satisfactions of this work among the dying are, as the nurse fresh from Vietnam remarked, very difficult, if not impossible, to describe. There is a great mystery in the power we experience, giving and receiving tenderness. And there is a mystery nearly glimpsed, nearly understood at moments, in being with people young or old who are very close to death. The usual walls and barriers of our own perception have a way of crumbling quietly, very nearly vanishing in such situations; "failing" no longer has anything whatever to do with *failure;* and by participating fully in the reality of dying, we ourselves find that we have learned better how to live. "I see everything so differently now," said a hospice nurse from the PCS in Montreal. "Colors, flowers, grass, things I never used to notice, all look so fresh and so amazing. Even the air smells different. God, it is all so beautiful!"

So it is for each one of us, living and dying, when the usual systems of our elaborate defenses are stripped away. Castle walls protect, but they also keep us prisoners under protection from all the wonders that lie beyond. Some of those wonders are very simple indeed, and may be seen at hand by anyone willing to make a profession of looking for them. Where the fortress fails, wildflowers soon spring up, bees follow gathering their nectar, and among ruins, often in the most unlikely crevices of all, birds come to build the small, round hallows of their nests.

Greatest of Feasts

CHAPTER 12

Love reveals more than hope can, for love is a mystical possessing *now* of all that hope looks for in the future.

George Congreve, S.S.J.E.

Again and again throughout these pages, the image of journeying recurs; and the writing of them has been in itself a kind of journey, a search not only for facts, but for meanings: the shapes and forms that invisible energies take in our lives. To journey is to move, to grow, to be in process, transforming what we see and hear and touch along the way, and experiencing the mystery of our own transformation. Material things and events are devoured by our senses, becoming the stuff of the mind, energetic and magnetic, that is the means, the fuel—and the map, as well—of our constant thrusting and voyaging into the unknown. Often, the traveler does not know what he is seeking until he has found it; and the pilgrim's goal in the end, whatever its symbolic form may be, is never really a location or an object, but the achievement of a new state of being. *Pilgrim's Progress* is one way of telling the story; the epic of *Gilgamesh* from ancient Babylon is another. Dante's *Inferno* is a journey and a pilgrimage of transformation; so is the tale of St. George in Spenser's *Faërie Queene*. Princes and paupers made such journeys throughout the early folk tales and legends of our culture, seeking to find the secrets of their true being in the winning of new wisdom and the capture of a new level of consciousness. Arthurian knights sought wholeness in the vision of the Grail which could only be achieved by the pure in heart; and in Greek mythology, Jason and his mariners risked their earthly lives to gain powers of renewal in the form of the Golden Fleece. In China, Tao has been for centuries the Way of Enlightenment: the pilgrim's path and, at the same time, his ultimate goal. "I am the light of the world," said Jesus. "He that followeth me shall not walk in darkness, but shall have the light of life."

The great events of life, as we observe them, are still clearly recognizable as journeys: conception and birth, the various places of passage such as puberty, entrance into adulthood, work and creation, marriage and generativity, maturity, old age. The invention of a new device or concept is the result of a voyage of the mind and a return to port, ships laden. To learn a new skill is to dare a movement toward growth, and in the very process of daring it, to grow. Prayer and meditation are journeys; so is the making of a poem or the composition of a symphony. To fall in love, as we all know, is to experience a stunning process of movement and change; and to explore that love over a period of many years is both a journey and a transformation.

It is not surprising, given the persistence of such realizations by people in so many lands and ages, to find that dying has also been seen throughout human history as a process of journeying. The understanding of death as one in a series of quite natural, though ultimately mysterious, personal transformations is so common among members of the human race that it could almost be called a definitive trait of our species. There are exceptions to this rule, of course. Entire societies get trapped from time to time in a sort of grey, empty space of confusion about the facts of death; and this happens most often when the current state of scientific knowledge appears to contradict the larger body of experience on which we base our sense of what is true. Western attitudes toward death and dying have obviously suffered in the past century or so from a period of such confusion. And at almost any time, a group or a tribe can be found tucked away in the hills of some primitive land, where death is seen as an assault on human dignity and a cosmic outrage. To the Juiraros, for example, a tribe dwelling in recent years on the eastern slopes of the Andes:

... there is no such thing as a natural death. While they may realize that death is a separation of body and spirit, they cannot seem to understand the general relation of natural causes to it. Each death to them is unintelligible, unnatural and accidental.... Since every death is presumably a murder, great excitement results. This is evidenced by the beating of the signal drums. ...

In civilized western society, sirens and telephones serve as our signal drums. Frightened and outraged, feeling defeated by death, we forget the ancient wisdom that is our heritage and that is, even today, being returned to us by a new set of observations.

Navajo Indians, curiously enough, are one of the few cultural groups in the world ever to have taken the position that there is no life whatever after death. Individuals, of course, have always appeared with intellectual systems designed along such lines; but societies as a whole have believed otherwise, and have passed down to succeeding generations the observation that something leaves the body at the moment of death, and seems to enter another form or level of existence. The Navajo groups who denied this found it very difficult to deal with the consequences of their denial; and their management of death and dying in such circumstances is interesting in comparison with our own, in conventional medical situations today.

The seriously ill Indian was carried away from his own *hogan* and isolated from all but one or two members of the tribe who stayed, waiting in dread for him to die. Silence was the rule when death did come; no mourning or mention of the event was considered appropriate. Quickly then, the body and all personal possessions of the deceased, including his *hogan*, were burned and the ashes were buried out of sight. So powerful was the need to deny the reality of death in these groups, that the person who had stayed with the dying, and performed these final rites, was shunned afterward as *taboo*. Death was the end, it was consciously believed, and thus was too terrible an event to be admitted into the process of tribal existence. Yet in such a situation, death is obviously not the end after all; for death itself in such a society has to be dealt blow after blow in a ritualized attempt to kill it. It is life that dies, under such circumstances, while death lives on.

Our own defense mechanisms on the subject represent just such a ritualistic defeat of conscious purpose. Yet, we do have a choice. We can dare a new point of view, and in daring it, can change. In the presence of death we can make the decision to stay open, not to draw back in dismay from the person who is dying, not to shun (on the excuse of embarrassment, but really in dread) the bereaved; and not to defend ourselves foolishly against the demanding realities of the mourning process. And if we care to place any trust in the vast accumulation of humanity's knowledge of the subject, and informed belief about it, we can stay open to the experience of our own dying, with the sense that it will be in some way a familiar journey, not unlike the journey of being born.

"My bags are packed," said Pope John in 1965, "I am ready to go." This has been the attitude, not only of the wise, the elderly, and the religious throughout human history; not only of the mystics, poets, and prophets of every age; but of countless millions of simple, practical people who have "watched and waked" at the deathbeds of friends and parents, spouses and children, who have held these dying people in their arms, looking straight into their eyes, hearing their last words and noticing closely what was happening to them. "The old folk . . . Russians, Tartars, Votyaks . . . didn't puff themselves up or fight against it . . . they prepared themselves quietly and in good time. . . . and they departed easily, as if they were just moving into a new house," writes Solzhenitsyn. "But 'tis the way, lad Kerry," says the ancient wise woman of the village in Donn Byrne's *Destiny Bay*. "Dying is like a boy's voice breaking and his putting on trews, or like a young girl and she letting down the hem of her skirt and putting up her soft hair. . . . We are like childer on the floor, and the dead are grown up."

Out of centuries of experience has come the repeated observation that death appears to be a process rather than an event, a form of passage for human life which in some way continues to exist, journeying on. Rituals designed to respond appropriately to this view are in themselves life-enhancing, and among simple people are often as realistic and practical as their care of the dying has been. In the villages of Eastern Europe, for example, all doors and windows of the house have traditionally been thrown open immediately upon the death of an occupant, so that the spirit could move without hindrance into the life beyond. For the same purpose, holes were made in the rooftops of houses in rural Mexico. Ashanti tribes in Ghana have an ancient tradition of giving water at the very last to the dying, so that the thirsting spirit may climb more easily up the steep hill to eternity; a handkerchief is placed in the hands of the dead to wipe the sweat of this struggle into the world beyond. Buddhists in Japanese country villages sew a white pilgrim's garment for the body and put a bag of coins at its belt, so that the departing spirit can pay the ferryman for its passage into eternity. Villagers in Moslem Turkey leave a light burning forty days and nights after a death, in the belief that the newly released soul may need its help in the process of learning to live without a physical body.

Death as a form of liberation is a motif familiar throughout the cultures of the world. In India the *Shraddha* ceremony is performed by Hindus to help the spiritual body to its celestial abode; death is perceived as the moment of freedom when this final journey can begin. The *Cho-Hon* ceremony in Korea represents an "Invitation to the Soul" in this stage of its pilgrimage; and *sajas* (like the spiritual companions seen at the last by modern patients of Dr. Elisabeth Kübler-Ross) are the messengers who come to guide it on its way. Viking chieftains who died were sent out to sea in their ships with all their possessions on board for the journey to the afterlife, and the ships were then set ablaze to help the spirit free itself from the last of its material bonds. These are universal responses to a mystery, a process in human life which has been observed over the ages by people in wholly contrasting cultures as essentially the same: a journey toward the liberation that exists beyond time and space. The following words might have been written by a poet or a prophet from any one of these ancient cultures; actually, they are the utterance of a modern German, Dietrich Bonhoeffer, who was imprisoned at the time, and later executed, by Adolf Hitler:

> Come now, thou greatest of feasts on the
>   journey to freedom eternal;
> Death, cast aside all the burdensome chains,
>   and demolish
> The walls of our temporal body, the walls of
>   our souls that are blinded
> So that at last we may see that which here
>   remains hidden.
> Freedom, how long have we sought thee in
>   discipline, action and suffering;
> Dying, we now behold thee revealed in
>   the Lord.

Fed on this part of our journey by our five senses and by all the beauties and gratifications of this world, we are aware still of being imprisoned by the limitations of ego, and we hunger for something beyond. Mystics have taught us for centuries that spirit takes only a temporal, restricted form in us while we dwell on earth; and that our five senses continually blunder, misinforming us and distracting our gaze from the essence of life which is holy and eternal. Time and space, they have insisted, should not be taken in the way we perceive them here and now, as practical measures of truth. Mystics are unpopular, however, in a world full of technological marvels and material riches. As consumers of such goods they are strangely lax and disinterested; the signs and symbols of worldly power habitually fail to impress them; and so "mystical" has gradually come to mean foggy and foolish, unrealistic, a little daft, maybe; and we have turned to the engineers, the technicians, and the scientists when we wanted firm truth.

Now, though, faced with a new set of scientific facts, it is we who sometimes must admit that we feel foggy and foolish.

Einstein teaches us that, for modern physicists, "this separation between past, present, and future has the value of mere illusion, however tenacious." Space, we are now told, somehow starts out more or less as we thought, then turns around and folds back into itself. What a poetic scientist has called "the gentle pressure of starlight" insists to our waking eyes that it is proceeding from a living, burning source; yet we know now that many of the stars we see above us went dark and died thousands upon thousands of years ago. Trying to deal with reality now, our scientists themselves are becoming poets and physicists are working in the realm of the metaphysical; once again we can all hear together the words of the mystics and the prophets such as T. S. Eliot, who writes:

> What we call the beginning is often the end
> And to make an end is to make a beginning . . .
> We shall not cease from exploration
> And the end of all our exploring
> Will be to arrive where we started
> And know the place for the first time . . .

To this Christian poet, dying is a process of transformation and transcendence continually happening during the measure of our earthly life. The journey of the soul toward God is a pilgrimage demanding that we strip away falsehood, pride, and the greedy demands of the ego so that we may move at last unencumbered, spiritually naked, in "A condition of complete simplicity/ (Costing not less than everything)" into the process of union with the divine. Glimpses of the goal are received along the way in a series of small deaths, moments of self-forgetfulness, worship and sacrifice which seem to stand beyond time, intersected by the flow of pure energy which is God's love. In this mode of perception, biological death can be understood as the annihilation of the final set of barriers between man and God, and as the supreme achievement of transcendence. Time does not matter here: "Before Abraham was," said Jesus, "I Am."

Images of blazing light appear very often in the attempts of seekers and religious mystics to describe these moments of dying to self and thus, moving beyond space and time. A sense of joy, unutterable peace and wholeness accompanies the unearthly radiance of this white light, which has been seen at such times and reported similarly, not only by poets such as Eliot and Blake, Wordsworth and Henry Vaughan ("I saw Eternity the other night/Like a great Ring of pure and endless light,/ All calm as it was bright . . ."); but also by ordinary people of various cultures and backgrounds studied in psychology texts, as William James' *The Varieties of Religious Experience*. Moses saw such a light in the Burning Bush; and Saul was temporarily blinded by it, on the road to Damascus. The disciplines of the Oriental sages are often built on an attempt to slip from the bondages of daily life and achieve this same sort of vision; and in fact, our way of expressing any sudden attainment of superior knowledge and wisdom is based on it, for we speak, not only in esoteric circles of "achieving enlightenment" but in plain language, of "seeing the light."

It is not so remarkable, perhaps, to find a matching set of experiences among seeking and journeying people in a number of different cultures, as it is to discover that these very same experiences are now being described by individuals who have clinically "died" and then, on account of modern resuscitation techniques, have recovered. Research by Elisabeth Kübler-Ross, reports them and more are documented by Raymond A. Moody, Jr. (*Life After Life*, Atlanta, 1975) in the cases of 150 people who had been very close to death or who, having been pronounced biologically dead, later "came back to life." All report the experience of dying as something like a journey, a movement out of space and time in an indescribable spiritual body "like an energy, maybe" or as one person put it, "something I can best describe as an energy pattern." Like Kübler-Ross's patients, Moody's subjects very often reported the presence of spiritual companions during this part of the dying process, and they also told of going through dark, tunnel-like spaces on their way toward the brilliance of the light. Then came emergence into tremendous radiance and joy, in the presence of a "being of light" whose love for them was overwhelming and indescribable:

> I floated . . . up into this pure crystal clear light, an illuminating white light. It was beautiful and so bright, so radiant, but it didn't hurt my eyes. It's not any kind of light you can describe on earth. I didn't actually see a person in this light, and yet it has a special identity, it definitely does. . . .

said one subject. And, another;

> I was out of my body, there's no doubt about it, because I could see my own body there on the operating room table. My soul was out! All this made me feel very bad at first, but then, this really bright light came . . . It was tremendously bright; I just can't describe it . . . Yet from the moment the light spoke to me, I felt really good—secure and loved. The love which came from it is just unimaginable, indescribable. It was a fun person to be with! And it had a sense of humor, too—definitely!

Religious people tended to describe this "being of light" as an angel, Jesus, or God; and even firm atheists, Dr. Moody reports, perceived it as some sort of religious figure. On returning from these journeys, as all his subjects obviously did, they felt powerfully changed by them, lifted to new levels of consciousness and committed to a set of values in which things of the mind and spirit took new precedence over the merely material. Many felt commanded by the experience to work toward a personal transformation which would allow them to love others on earth as they in their "time out of time" had felt loved. Though Moody himself makes no judgment of these cases and merely reports them as they occurred, it seems reasonable to state here that these were experiences of personal transformation, conversion and spiritual growth.

In a recent interview (*McCalls*, August 1976), Dr. Kübler-Ross reports a typical case of her own. The patient was a thirty-nine year old man near death after a massive coronary:

"He experienced himself floating out of his body toward a beckoning light. He said later that he felt that if he had gone much closer to the light he would not have returned to his body . . ."

"And what is the light?" the interviewer asked.

"That light is God," Dr. Kübler-Ross replied, in total earnestness. "God is the light and love these people experience. They are entering His presence. That, for me, is beyond the shadow of a doubt."

This patient then heard the voices of his young children (who were not present at the time) crying for him and realized that he must return to life to take care of them; and many of Dr. Kübler-Ross's and Raymond Moody's subjects experienced similar "recalls," sensing that they must go back, or that they were being sent back to fulfill their responsibilities, by the "being of light." In the experiences of most, the matter of responsibility did not end with "dying," in fact. There followed, in the presence of the light, a miraculously rapid review of the actions and events of the person's entire life. This resembled the Judgment in ancient Egyptian and in medieval Christian traditions except that it was done in a wholly loving and accepting way, demonstrating mistakes with the sense that one should learn from them to comprehend more and do better. The individual then returned to ordinary existence feeling in some way reborn.

Symbolically, we perform rites of this sort, or rites allowing for this sort of experience to take place, when we undergo religious disciplines of fasting or meditation and when we baptize, recognizing that new birth and transformation cannot take place without a letting-go of ego which is a sort of death. The Judgment appears in various dramatic forms in such ancient works as the Egyptian *Book of the Dead*, the Tibetan *Bardo Thödol* and the medieval Christian work, *The Craft of Dying (Ars Moriendi)*; and all agree that the state of mind of the dying person is of utmost importance to his ultimate destiny. Many of the experiences reported by subject of modern research appear in very similar form in the works of 2,000 years ago; differences seem to be mainly cultural and, interestingly enough, connected with differing ideas about the purpose of human life in its relation to space and time. All see death as a form of journey. The description of the process in the "secret" Tibetan book, which until recent years was unavailable except to the initiate, is very complicated and its imagery is so unfamiliar to the western reader that most of us must begin with Carl Jung's explanation of it and then go for help to someone who can explain to us the explanation of Dr. Jung. But of course, this is the reason why it is so fascinating to see the same perceptions turning up in parallel forms, in the experiences of modern Americans.

Tibetans teach that the dying person will see, at the moment when life ceases, almost immediately a brilliant light. He will go through a series of struggles after this which represent various levels of spiritual development coming under attack from negative forces of worldly temptation. Escape from the almost certain fate of reincarnation (perhaps in some lower form) can only be achieved by resisting all of these illusions and entering at last, in the ecstatic state known as *Samadhi,* into the Clear Light of the Void. The esoteric *Bardo Thödol* is a sort of instruction book for the newly dead, and is supposed to be recited by the person's spiritual guide for a period of many days so that, in all the confusion of the passage, its wisdom will not be forgotten. Medieval Christians in *Ars Moriendi,* not believing in the possibility of reincarnation, felt that such spiritual counseling must take place as the person was dying, and emphasized the necessity for confession of sins and death of egoistic desires before the individual should come into the immediate presence of God. Both agreed, however, that "to know how to die is to know how to live," and that these spiritual teachings should be a part of the daily life of all who sought enlightenment.

Both agreed too, along with most other major religious groups in the world, that the manner of death is deeply significant (suicide, for example, being seen as extremely destructive, if not fatal to the soul) and that the care of the dying was a delicate matter to be handled by the yogi, the priest, or the elder with great powers of spiritual authority. As the delightfully forthright little volume *Ars Moriendi* puts it,

> When any of likelihood shall die, then it is most necessary to have a special friend, the which will heartily help and pray for him and therewith counsel the sick for the weal of his soul; and moreover to see that all others do so about him or else quickly for to make them depart.

Right dying, Tibetan sages say, is an initiation. Therefore this is a process that should happen consciously. *Ars Moriendi* agrees, and gives the example of Isaiah the Prophet:

> For when the King Ezechiel lay sick and upon the point of death, he glosed him not, nor used no dissimulation unto him, but plainly and wholesomely aghasted him, saying that he should die.

The idea of "wholesomely aghasting" someone on his deathbed was to make certain that he got ready for his journey "up Godward" at this time of passage. But the wise man lived all his life in a Godward direction and was not distracted by the illusory successes or failures, pleasures, or terrors of this world any more than the obedient Tibetan was, by the demons and the visions of the world below. The ultimate goal of union with God is the same in both traditions, and the fact that East and West have tended to disagree on how long this takes and where it happens becomes relatively insignificant in view of the fact that both disciplines aim to help the individual out of space and time, into eternity.

"Is There an Answer to Death?" inquires the title of a recent book on the subject, which has suddenly become so popular, of death and dying. To this perhaps we had best reply, as Gertrude Stein is said to have done on her own deathbed, "What was the question?" Bumbling around as we are in a universe so complex that we may only glimpse once or twice in a lifetime, at best, any really intelligent question to ask about it, we are not very likely to seize on a system here, in the midst of the twentieth century, which will control all our future thinking about death and dying in an acceptable fashion. Our present attempts have got to be modest and ought to contain—like the Being of Light many have perceived—a very definite sense of humor; for we should keep in mind the sort of equipment we are using when we try to grapple with these ultimate issues. As geneticist Francois Jacob reminds us:

> This evolutionary procedure—the formation of a dominating neocortex coupled with the persistence of a nervous and hormonal system partially, but not totally under the rule of the neocortex . . .is somewhat like adding a jet engine to an old horse cart.

It is a tinkerer's universe, Jacob says, made of structures put together with odd bits and pieces of whatever was lying around. If so, then it is a poet's and a prophet's universe as well, where metaphor is a handy tool for the geneticist describing it. The jet engine causes the old horse cart no end of trouble, heaving it hither and yon until it splits its seams at last, casting cargo over the landscape and ending up abandoned by the side of the road. Perhaps this is why there is so often a sense of terror associated with the highest functions of this new energy ("Go, go, go said the bird: human kind/Cannot bear very much reality"), and perhaps this is why we, the living, think of dying as such a frightening catastrophe. Something in us wants to be pure energy, without even the casings of a jet. Throughout our lives we grope toward a goal that feels to some like personal liberation and to others, like union with the divine. Religious people of most cultures would say that it is both, and that the agent of all our transformations along the way is that "being of light" which is called by so many of us, God.

To those of us who are concerned today to find better ways of caring for the dying, both Eastern and Western traditions have much to teach us; and those who have worked with patients in the modern hospice situation can confirm the view of both, that the process of dying offers tremendous potential for personal growth. In the caring community of a hospice, the individual is provided with the kind of time and space that does not concern itself with worldly status or the winning of any war, but only with the process of pure being, as it is acted out in the giving and receiving of human love. Those who do hospice work, whatever the structure of their religious or philosophical beliefs, tend to feel for this reason that there is a sort of centeredness and holiness about it. Whether they are offering massage or medicine for pain, clean linens, or a hand to hold and a listening heart, they sense that these are gestures of obedience to Love of higher order. And the dying who are cared for in this way are offered, without any preaching or intellectualizing about it, a clear representation of that "time out of time" which is celebrated by our poets and our prophets, and in our liturgies.

What are the strange journeys of the Egyptians and the Tibetans in their Underworlds, and the voyages of the dead or dying people studied in modern times? I am not sure that it matters very much whether these people were clinically dead or clinically alive when they had these experiences, though the borderlines of our judgments about clinical death may shift somewhat as a result of such observations. This is not what proves to me that there is something eternal in life, and something holy. What seems to me important about these journeys is the sense of bliss, of sudden understanding, and of arrival in the blazing presence of Love, which is the same experienced in the "small deaths" of ritual, prophecy, and poetry. To be at home in the universe is to be a pilgrim, and yet not a stranger. A kind of space is required for this, in which we can change and grow while being welcomed in all our transformations. The hospice offers this kind of space to the dying. Time is insignificant in this setting except as it serves the needs of the patient's awareness. Space is ordered here in such a way that bodily discomforts do not distract, and the mind and the soul can roam at their ease, unconfined. Heaven indeed is open (as they believed in sixteenth century Spain) to the dying who are received and welcomed in the hospice community;

and here they are offered by the disintegration of the material body, a richer matrix than ever for spirit to grow in.

To those of us who are witness to such events, the phrase "Life after Death" tends to become inadequate to the experience, if not altogether irrelevant. Lillian Preston did not begin to live until she reached the time and the place where she lay dying. In a garden in Charleston in the spring, Miss Aurelia Robbins still walks under the curving glass of time, sheltered among her lilies and her snowflakes, blind and smiling and so very, very grateful in her soft, white dress. To have known these people—and Mr. Pippin, and Mrs. Doe, and Jim Burham, the young musician—is to have experienced in the here and now a kind of immutable wholeness, and holiness.

"Let me tell you, Doctor," said an 83-year-old Hospice of Marin patient recently, "dying is the experience of a lifetime." What she meant by these splendid words remains, like the very fabric of life itself, a mystery. "I think I was meant to come here," says Lillian Preston's final letter from St. Christopher's Hospice, "so that at last, I could experience joy." Caring and being cared for in such an environment, she was transformed. To have lived in the hospice community, to have watched and waked with the dying throughout these pages has been for me as well, a journey of personal transformation. The people I have come to know here are part of me now; and those who have left on the longer journey before me have brought, in their caring for me, a great part of me with them. Together, living and dead, we now dwell in a place of eternal hospitality where there is no before and no after—there is only love.

A Personal Afterword

Female, single, Caucasian, age 47—and in a general hospital, because there was no hospice unit available yet to receive her—on Midsummer's Eve of this year, my friend Anne died.

It had been a long struggle: cancer of the esophagus; then, after the most delicate and skillful of surgical intervention, a sudden, explosive spread of malignancy throughout her body. Like the woman whose name I will never know who died beside me years ago, Anne was fated to fight a large part of her battle alone. In her case, however, this was for a time a matter of personal choice. Anne was private as a cat, fastidious, aloof and quixotic to the point of eccentricity. I loved her. Many people did not. She was proud, quick-tempered, wrote odd poems, painted watercolors no one wanted to buy. She quarreled regularly with her neighbors over such matters as disappearing trashbin tops and dogs that barked in the night. Anne was "difficult"—a determined loner—and though few people knew it, by the end of her long illness, she was quite literally destitute.

Yet despite all this, and despite the fact that our community's hospice unit may not be ready for another year, Anne did not die in despair, a surgical-chemical cripple automatically overtreated, then abandoned as a medical "failure" at the last. She did not die screaming, calling out for help. The final days of her life were filled with loving-kindness given and received, with moments of wonder and of humor, a new sort of openness, trust and tenderness about her; and at the end, the huge, dark eyes that seemed by then almost all that was left of her gazed quite clearly, with fierce curiosity, into the unknown.

Under the circumstances, it was a makeshift sort of miracle that happened. Nevertheless it did occur, and it served to remind those of us who witnessed it that *hospice,* at base, is not a new form of magic, but an ancient and sensible, decent form of human behavior. Anne's death was proof that hospitality can be brought to bear in the most difficult of situations, if only people understand what it is, and are willing to work for it.

It would have been better, of course, if Anne could have died in the quiet simplicity of the hospice facility we dream of now and work for daily. As it was, she died owing—and being owed—debts both financial and emotional that can never be repaid. She should have died, if not in a hospice unit, then in her own little garden, watching her hummingbirds at their feeder—they were her greatest joy. She should have died hearing her favorite Mozart and Vivaldi, instead of the loudspeakers in the hospital repeating their litanies of panic, day and night, down echoing corridors. Anne loved fresh air, polished pebbles, feathers, the smell of the herbs she grew in other people's cast-off, broken pots, the slant of the morning light in the little studio-apartment where she painted, almost to the end, intensely shy and cautious renderings of leaves, buds, birds and shells. Her ward in the hospital smelled of disinfectant, pus and fear. No sun came in. Toward the end I thought more than once of carrying her away from there, bundling her out under a cloak or in a laundry bag. She was so small and frail by then, I could have done it. Her suitcase, when I carried it away for her later, was far heavier. But, where. . .? And who would help with the kind of care she needed? There was no hospice building waiting to welcome her.

There was, however, a hospice team forming in our neighborhood just then; and part of the miracle was that several of its members had already become acquainted with Anne, over the years. As her illness progressed, we discovered that she was willing to share a part of her life with us that she badly needed to conceal from the rest of the world. Anne had been taught young to despise weakness. Seeing that we did not, she did not feel ashamed to show herself, as she was, to us. Day by day growing more needy and more helpless, she drew a circle—a very small one—of "hospice people" around her, and in doing so, brought us closer to one another. Dying, she helped to create community.

Anne's physician, though not formally a member of the hospice group, was aware and sympathetic: a sensitive human being as well as a fine medical man. When he had done all that was possible to combat the malignancy, he did not turn away. He focused his attention not upon cancer, the disease, but upon Anne, the person. Pain was not a major problem in her case, and so she did not need the help of a Hospice Mix. Discomforts there were, however, and these her physician noted and negotiated constantly, directing her nursing care so that Anne could have every possible relief. Feeding, which she emphatically rejected toward the end, was never forced. Oxygen was available as she needed it, but machinery was not applied to coerce her lungs; and in her final hours, Anne was not isolated from the presence of those she had chosen to draw together in the intimacy of a family circle. Visiting rules, as far as we were concerned, were quietly eliminated. We came to her when she wanted us—or when we sensed that she wanted us—separately and together, feeling our way, learning as best we could from her day by day, moment by moment toward the end, how we might help.

Nurses and aides meantime came and went on their various shifts—how seldom we ever saw the same one twice! Some of these were disinterested, perfunctory; but others, both young and old, were tender and sensitive, noticing our presence with grateful eyes, asking us questions about hospice work, and slipping in quietly from time to time during their busy rounds to join our circle at Anne's bedside.

At the very end, a telephone call came across the country for Anne, from a man she loved. The hospice team had located him that day, and had let him know that the end was near; but in the meantime the central switchboard had been told, no more calls for her, it was too late. Technically, of course, it was. Anne was by now far too weak to lift a telephone, even to speak. But in the temporary absence of the hospice group, it was one of the noticing, questioning nurses who intervened. Understanding what must be done for Anne, she fought the switchboard and rerouted the call. Then, holding Anne in her arms and the telephone close to her ear, she stood by until the last words were spoken, so that Anne was able to hear at the very moment of her death, in the beloved voice, "Anne, I love you."

A small miracle, but a real one. And an important one because, unlike cancer, the hospice point of view is definitely contagious. Wherever it goes, if its intent is clearly stated, it will tend to work its gently, stubbornly persuasive way. Within the hospital its presence brings subtle changes that will help to alter our entire society's attitudes about death, and about those who are dying. With separate hospices appearing as communities-within-community in the years to come, its healing transformations will come about even more rapidly. People like Anne will not feel such a desperate need to hide themselves away; and those of us who are newly enabled to receive the dying into our midst will be helped to accept from them their very real, very great gifts.

It seems appropriate for me now, having admitted my strong prejudice in favor of free-standing hospice inpatient units, to end this book with Anne's story, in a hospital. For it is entirely clear by now that mere architecture, however pleasing, cannot make a hospice; and that true hospice care cannot be artificially programmed. Care is care. It is not a building, a grant, a law, or a committee. *Remember Anne,* I think, when I hear of hospice committees now across the country studying other hospice committees, or calling in "outside planners"—presumably to make elaborate and expensive outside plans of all that has not been happening inside. This is not hospice work; this is mere fiddling and politics. Hospice work does not begin with charts of administrative functions, or lists of potential sites, or willing benefactors. Hospice work begins with the question, *What does this patient need?*

Anne needed a great deal that we were unable to give her. The place she died in was wrong for her, the tempo was not right, the confusion of constantly shifting personnel hurt her, the sounds she heard and the very air she breathed were debilitating and distracting to one in her condition. Yet even in Anne's situation, a kind of healing was possible. Seeing day by day that she was acceptable to our small group, that we honored her no matter how she looked or felt or behaved at the moment, Anne, who had always been so withdrawn, began to reveal a hidden side of her character. All this time, we discovered, she had wanted very much to care for other people and, like many who are equally shy and aloof, had a secretly passionate need to be needed.

Our reaction to this, we realized in talking together later, had been—at the time of her great physical and emotional weakness—to let her see that we quite honestly depended on her, valued her advice, needed her support as individuals and, as a developing group, were nourished by her encouragement. Some of us told her now, for the first time, our personal troubles, somewhat as travelers tend to confide sudden intimacies to the stranger who will be leaving the train or the ship at its next stopping place. Illness had aged Anne's face, stripped it bare of all but wisdom and nobility, so that huddled in her little chair in the garden, and later, in her hospital bed, she seemed at times like the ancient crone in the forests of mythology, who gives the seeker a password or a magic token that will help him find his way. As her body withered, her spirit blazed more fiercely, her wit grew sharper, and her words—measured out now by the claims of physical weakness—were more profound and simple, wise and direct.

Four nights before she died, Anne achieved a major personal triumph. Private in her ways as she had always been, she felt deeply the trespass and insult of lying side by side with other patients, having her bodily functions casually placed on view, and being forced to witness the intimacies of others. On this night in June, a large, black, middle-aged woman, sobbing and wailing, was placed in the bed next to Anne's "for observation" after an automobile accident. Anne learned from the nurses' talk that the woman's only child had been burned to death in the crash that afternoon, and that the woman's condition in all probability was "just emotional." The woman was given sedation, told to go to sleep, and hastily left to lie alone in the dark with her grief. Anne was furious. Although she had been too weak for several days to take any nourishment, or even to sit up in bed, she somehow managed to clamber down to the floor, crawled on bare knees across the intervening space, and pulled herself up to embrace her sobbing neighbor. In the hour that followed, the dying tended the living in a way that no professional person present had thought to do. Six months earlier, I doubt that Anne could have done it herself. Shyness and scorn for her own grief, as well as the grief of others, would have held her back. As it was, Anne transformed herself into an active hospice worker before she died.

"*Not dying,*" she informed John, our hospice chaplain, in no uncertain terms when he arrived for his usual afternoon visit, on the last day. She knew perfectly well what was happening to her. But by now John and Anne had established a relationship filled with mischief and bantering—that was their mode. John took her hand and held it. "Anne, my dear, you are very, very sick and you know it," he said to her sternly, with a twinkle in his eye.

"*So?*" she replied with a wicked grin, and closed her eyes, content. As far as she was concerned, she had won that round. Three of us stood around her bed then, looking at one another, caught between laughter and tears. Anne had been moved to a sort of utility space, windowless, curtained off, out of sight. In a moment she took up her conversation with John again in a perfectly normal tone but in words, suddenly, that none of us could understand. Her hands were like shells to hold, so fragile, cool, and dry. There was so much she wanted to tell us. She talked and talked, mystery.

"What can we do for you, Anne?" asked the chaplain and then, seeing her moving away from us so quickly, called after her louder, "Anne, what can we do?"

"Stay," she whispered. We did. She was quiet for a time, then opened her eyes, looked from one to the other of us and firmly commanded us, "Pray."

Loudspeakers blared, calling for doctors, as John anointed her forehead with the holy oil. She smiled up at him, whispering . . . something. A joke? Gurneys rattled by. "That's how Joshua smelled at the Battle of Jericho, Anne," said John. She smiled again, words tumbling out endlessly; she was trying with the last of her strength, it seemed, to tell us what it was like for her now, where she was going, what she was seeing, wanting to bring us with her, letting us know it was curious—bewildering—amazing—but yes, all right. "For I am persuaded," John was saying, "that neither death nor life, nor angels, nor principalities nor powers, nor things present, nor things to come, nor height, nor depth nor anything created can separate us from the love of God. . ." and to these radiant words of Paul's Epistle, Anne responded instantly with words of her own, incomprehensible, passionate, magnificent. She saw something then that the rest of us may have glimpsed at moments, opened her eyes, started to speak—and then did not, assuming, obviously, that we could see it too. In her garden one morning early, with almost the same strange smile she had said to me, "Look!" and made a puzzle out of it, a treasure hunt. At last I understood that day, it was the hummingbirds. She had just put up their feeder, and they had found it. "Their wings," she said. "Look, look, their wings move so fast, you can't really see them. Yet, they are there."

When I think of her now, I sometimes see her in the garden as she was that day, but even more clearly as she lay looking up at us in the hospital, utterly certain that we too had found the treasure and were rejoicing with her in the glory of it—the incredible ease, and the wit. Happiness is not the word to describe the look on her face at that moment, nor is peace. Joy is not strong enough. There was humor in it, and rapture—and something even beyond. Perhaps Anne gave up speaking to us after this, even in her own private language, for such reasons: There was nothing more to say. We thought a few moments later that she had fallen asleep, but she had not. She was waiting for her telephone call.

Remember Anne.

Author's Note:

Readers wishing further information about hospices presently forming or operating in the U.S.A. are advised to contact:

National Hospice Organization
c/o Dennis Rezendes
765 Prospect Street
New Haven, CT 06511

Drug Control of Common Symptoms

APPENDIX A

St. Christopher's Hospice

PAIN CONTROL

More than 60 percent of patients admitted to St. Christopher's Hospice complain of pain: sometimes mild, often severe, not infrequently overwhelming. All these patients subsequently experience substantial, if not complete, relief.

Perhaps the two most important reasons for inadequate pain control prior to admission are:

- An inadequate concept of the nature of pain.
- Ill-founded fears and fantasies concerning the "addictive" nature of narcotic analgesics.

Pain due to advancing cancer is usually chronic, constant in nature even if variable in intensity. Chronic pain, unlike acute pain, is a situation rather than an event. It is impossible to predict when it will end; it usually gets worse rather than better; it appears to be entirely meaningless and, often, expands to occupy the patient's whole attention, isolating him from the world around. Depression, anxiety, fear, mental isolation, other unrelieved symptoms, and pain itself will tend to exacerbate the total pain experience. To relieve such pain all these factors must be considered.

Addiction—a compulsion or overpowering drive to take a drug in order to experience its psychological effects—does not occur when patients' pain control is part of a pattern of total care. Occasionally a patient admitted to the Hospice appears to be addicted, demanding "an injection" every two or three hours. Such a patient typically has a long history of poor pain control and will, for several weeks, have been receiving fairly regular ("four-hourly prn") but inadequate injections of one or more narcotic analgesics. Given time, it is usually possible to control the pain, prevent clock-watching and demanding behavior and, sometimes, transfer the patient to an oral preparation. But even here, can it be said that the patient is really addicted? Is he craving the narcotic in order to experience its psychological effects? Or is he craving relief from pain, in part if not in full, for at least an hour or two?

Analgesics should be given regularly, usually four-hourly. The aim is to titrate the level of analgesia against the patient's pain, gradually increasing the dose until the patient is pain-free, the next dose being given before the effect of the previous one has worn off and therefore before the patient may think it necessary. In this way it is possible to erase the memory and fear of pain.

If a rapid increase in dose is required to maintain an adequate level of analgesia, additional or alternative measures should be considered; for example, an anti-inflammatory agent (such as phenylbutazone or prednisolone) or radiotherapy if the pain is due to skeletal metastases; a phenol nerve block if due to nerve compression. When the dose has to be increased fairly rapidly the patient may at first feel sleepy but tolerance to the sedative effect of narcotic analgesics and phenothiazines usually occurs within two or three days.

Mild Pain

1. Paracetamol (Panadol): 2 four-hourly
2. Dextropropoxyphene with paracetamol (Distalgesic): 2 four-hourly.
3. Soluble Aspirin: 2 four-hourly or Codis: 2 four-hourly.

These are also used as adjuncts to stronger analgesics and are often useful in bone pain and headache.

Moderate Pain

1. Dipipanone 10 mg with cyclizine 30 mg (Diconal); 1-2 four-hourly (tab 1 equivalent to 2.5-5 mg diamorphine). This is a useful analgesic of medium strength and is especially valuable with outpatients or if the patient prefers a tablet to a mixture.

2. Diamorphine and cocaine elixir: (see note below)

      Diamorphine Hcl 5-10 mg—increasing as necessary

      Cocaine 10 mg

      Chloroform water to 10 ml

Unless transferring from another potent narcotic analgesic, the initial dose given is usually 5 mg (2.5 mg may be sufficient for the frail and elderly). This is given with a phenothiazine, often as a syrup. Prochlorperazine (Stemetil) 5 mg in 5 ml is the one usually added, chlorpromazine (Largactil) 12.5-25 mg in 5 ml if sedation is required. These potentiate the effect of diamorphine, and also act as anti-emetics and tranquilizers. For outpatients, Stemetil or Largactil Syrup can be incorporated in the mixture when a stable level of analgesia is obtaind, e.g.:

      Diamorphine Hcl   20 mg

      Cocaine   10 mg

      Stemetil Syrup   5 ml

      Chloroform Water to 10 ml

The diamorphine and cocaine elixir BPC may be used; it contains 5 mg diamorphine and 5 mg cocaine in a 5 ml dose. The disadvantage is that, if the analgesic needs to be increased, then the dose of cocaine and the volume to be taken will be increased proportionally.

3. Phenazocine (Narphen): 5 mg 1-3 four-hourly (5 mg equivalent to 10-15 mg diamorphine).

This is a useful strong analgesic, especially if the patient dislikes the diamorphine and cocaine elixir, or prefers a tablet.

Note: See Chapter 6 note *re:* recent substitution of morphine for diamorphine at St. Christopher's.

**Severe
Pain**

Diamorphine and cocaine elixir containing diamorphine 10–40 mg or even up to 80 mg four-hourly is
usually effective. If this does not control the pain with
the addition of adjuvants (e.g. Distalgesic: 2 four-
hourly) the patient should be transferred to four-hourly
injections of diamorphine, starting with one-half the
previous oral dose and increasing until the pain is
controlled.

The phenothiazine should continue to be given,
either orally or by injection. Diamorphine alone can be
given subcutaneously. However, for an exacerbation of
pain or a crisis no patient should be kept waiting for
relief.

**Pain
and
Vomiting**

The diamorphine and cocaine elixir with phenothiazine may be tolerated and prove effective.
However, it may be necessary to give injections of
diamorphine and a phenothiazine for a few days; this
may need to be prolonged in intractable vomiting,
obstruction, or if the patient cannot swallow; oxycodone pectinate (Proladone) suppositories (30 mg) 1–2
eight-hourly are occasionally used with outpatients to
avoid the regular injections of analgesics.

Bone Pain

This is a difficult problem, as frequently the pain
level varies widely and depends on the patient's
activity. It is often useful to add to analgesics an anti-
inflammatory agent. Aspirin is useful and phenylbutazone (Butazolidin or Butacote) will help about half
the patients. In severe bone pain phenylbutazone may
be started in a dosage of 600 mg–800 mg/day, reducing
after a week to 300 mg/day if possible. The drug should
be withdrawn if there is no improvement. Indomethacin (Indocid) and ibuprofen (Brufen) are probably
less potent alternatives.

**Other
Analgesics**

1. Morphine sulphate. A controlled double-blind
trial comparing morphine with diamorphine, given in
an elixir, showed that there was no clinically observable
difference (if given in the ratio of diamorphine: morphine = 1:1.5). There were no measurable differences

in side-effects, e.g., nausea, constipation, euphoria. However, diamorphine is still preferable if given by injection as it is much more soluble.

2. Methadone. This is probably equipotent with diamorphine but has a much longer half-life and therefore a cumulative effect which could be potentially dangerous in the very ill. It may be possible to give it less frequently, e.g., 6–8 hours.

ANOREXIA

This is one of the commonest symptoms in malignant disease. Glucocorticosteroids are frequently used, either prednisolone (enteric coated) 2.5 mg × 2 tds or prednisolone 5 mg tds. In the majority of cases this produces, after about a week, a marked increase in appetite and sense of well-being.

Alcohol before or with meals may help.

NAUSEA AND VOMITING

The phenothiazines are probably the most useful drugs. Prochlorperazine (Stemetil) 5–10 mg, promazine (Sparine) 25 mg or chlorpromazine (Largactil) 25 mg are all useful anti-emetics and are in ascending order of sedative effect.

They may be given four-hourly in syrup or as a suspension in the case of promazine (Sparine). Alternatively, they may be given in tablet form or by IM injection. Stemetil suppositories (25 mg) and Largactil suppositories (100 mg) are useful if oral preparations are not tolerated and injections impracticable—for example, if the patient is at home. These are normally given eight-hourly. If these prove inadequate it is probably better to add a further anti-emetic of a different type rather than to increase the dose. Cyclizine (Valoid) 50 mg orally or IM bd is often useful, as is metoclopramide (Maxolon) 10 mg, especially if given orally about one hour AC or IM.

Obstructive Vomiting

It is usually possible to control the pain and vomiting of malignant large bowel obstruction in its terminal phase by the use of adequate analgesics and combination of anti-emetics. In these cases Dioctyl-forte 1–2 tds are sometimes used until it appears that obstruction is complete. Lomotil 2 qds may have a place in the control of painful colic.

DRY MOUTH   This may be due to one or more of many causes, e.g., local radiotherapy, various drugs, dehydration. Intravenous fluids and nasogastric feeding cannot be justified in dying patients who rarely feel thirsty, and it is perfectly possible to correct the only common symptom of dehydration, namely, a dry mouth, by local measures such as frequent small drinks or crushed ice to suck.

HICCOUGH   Metoclopramide (Maxolon) 10 mg oral or IM.
Chlorpromazine (Largactil) 25 mg oral or IM.

DYSPNOEA   1. *Bronchodilators*
Salbutamol (Ventolin) 2–4 tds or Aminophylline suppositories 1–2 prn are used for bronchospasm.
2. *Glucocorticosteroids*
Prednisolone may help considerably when there is diffuse malignant involvement of the lungs and, of course, on bronchospasm. In such circumstances, the recommended starting dose is 10–15 mg tds, reducing gradually to 5 mg tds.
3. *Antibiotics*
If dyspnoea is associated with a cough productive of purulent sputum, an antibiotic may ease the patient's distress. But the indiscriminate use of antibiotics may merely prolong the terminal phase. Septrin, ampicillin, chloramphenicol are all used.
4. *Opiates*
In many cases, e.g., large pleural effusion and extensive carcinoma of bronchus, the above measures are ineffective and then opiates must be used to relieve the distress of continued dyspnoea. The diamorphine and cocaine elixir may be adequate, but more often injections or diamorphine are used with a phenpthiazine or diazepam (Valium) to combat the associated mental distress.
5. *Hyoscine*
IM hyoscine 0.4–0.6 mg is given with an opiate to

dry up the excessive secretions which accumulate when a patient is dying, and eliminates the "death rattle" which is distressing to relatives, if not to the patient.

NB: IM hyoscine with an opiate may give the quickest relief in a major crisis, e.g., haemorrhage or pulmonary embolus.

COUGH

1. Benylin Expectorant is often adequate
2. Linctus Methadone 5–10 ml, especially at night
3. Antibiotics
4. Bromhexine (Bisoivon) 8 mg tds (tao 1 or 10 ml syrup) is often effective in liquefyĩng tenacious sputum.
5. Diamorphine and cocaine elixir or injection given for pain or dyspnoea is, of course, also an effective cough suppressant.

ANXIETY, MENTAL DISTRESS

1. Diazepam (Valium) 2–5 tds
2. Promazine (Sparine) 25 tds or chlorpromazine (Largactil) 10–25 mg tds
3. IM or IV diazepam (Valium) 10 mg is of use in acute panic states or prior to some procedure which distresses the patient, e.g., a difficult catheterisation.

CONFUSION

In mild confusion oral chlorpromazine (Largactil) 10–25 mg qds may be adequate. In severe restlessness and confusion IM chlorpromazine (Largactil) 25–100 mg may be needed or IM methotrimaprazine (Veractil) 25–50 mg. These may be given with opiates or in conjunction with diazepam (Valium) if necessary. Thioridazine (Melleril) 10–25 mg has a place with the elderly.

DEPRESSION

1. Attention to physical and mental distress
2. Antidepressants

Tricyclic antidepressants, e.g., amitriptyline (Tryptizol) or trimipramine (Surmontil) either 10–25 mg tds or 25–50 mg nocte. Patients with malignant disease should usually be started on a small dose, e.g., 10 mg tds or 25 mg nocte as larger doses sometimes precipitate confusion. This is possibly due to their potentiation by the phenothiazines.

INSOMNIA   Non-barbiturate sedatives are preferred, dichloral-phenazone (Welldorm) or nitrazepam (Mogadon). It is sometimes useful to add chlorpromazine (Largactil) 25–50 mg either with the hypnotics or in the early evening. Chlormethiazole (Heminevrin) 500 mg–1G is useful in the elderly.

CONSTIPA-   Our patients do best with the combination of soften-
TION   ing and peristalsis-inducing aperients. Milpar 10 ml bd or Dioctyl-forte 1–2 tds, may be given with Senokot alternate nights; alternatively, a dual action preparation such as Dorbanex 1–2 bd or 5–10 ml bd. Glycerine suppositories may be needed, or a disposable phosphate enema.

   Bran is useful in the fairly small proportion of patients who can take it.

DIARRHOEA   1. Codeine phosphate 15–60 mg tds
   or
   2. Lomotil 2 qds.
   Some cases of diarrhoea are due to malabsorption from pancreatic insufficiency, and these respond to pancreatic replacements, e.g., caps Pancrex V 1 tds with food.

FUNGATING   1. Clean with Eusol and paraffin (1 part in 4) if
GROWTHS   offensive
   2. Antibiotic spray, e.g., Polybactrin, to combat local sepsis
   3. Non-adhesive dressing
   A course of systemic antibiotics may help to reduce sepsis with its associated offensive discharge.

FREQUENCY   1. Treatment of infection
   2. Emepronium bromide (Cetiprin) 100 mg tds or 200 nocte.

CATHETERISA- TION

1. Septrin 2 bd for two days when catheter is inserted or changed.
2. Maintenance on a urinary antiseptic, e.g., hexamine hippurate (Hiprex) 1 bd.
3. A course of an appropriate antibiotic should frank infection occur, as indicated by suprapubic pain, or if the catheter is blocked by debris.
4. Catheter changed every four weeks.
5. Regular bladder washouts with Hibitane 1 in 5,000, or Noxyflex bladder washouts bd for two days in patients unable to take urinary antiseptics by mouth or if, in spite of these, the catheter tends to block.

ITCH

1. Antihistamines, e.g., chlorpheniramine (Piriton) 4 mg tds
2. Steroids
3. In the irritation caused by biliary stasis cholestyramine (Cuemid, Questran) 1 sachet qds is the drug of choice, but patients find it difficult to take.
4. Crotamiton (Eurax) or local anaesthetic creams may be of value.

Reprinted here by permission of Dr. Cicely Saunders.

American Equivalents to Medicines in St. Christopher's Drug Chart

Appendix B

(Prepared by Donald T. Kishi, Pharm. D., Associate Clinical Professor of Pharmacy at the University of California, San Francisco)

Amitriptyline = Elavil[R]
Aspirin = Aspirin
Benylin Expectorant = Benylin[R] Expectorant
Bromhexine = Not available
              (An expectorant)
Chlormethiazole = Not available
              (Sedative-hypnotic with anticonvulsant effect)
Chlorpheniramine = Chlor-Trimeton[R]
Cholestyramine = Questran[R]
Codis = Codeine
Crotamiton = Eurax[R] Cream or Lotion
              (Antipruritic scabicide)
Cyclizine = Marezine[R]
Dextropropoxyphene with paracetamol = Darvon[R] with Tylenol[R]

Diamorphine = Heroin
Dichloralphenazone = Not available
                (Complex of chloral hydrate and
                phenazon)
Dioctyl Forte = Doss = Colace[R]
Dipipanone with cyclizine
  Dipipanone = Piperidyl Methadone = Not available
  Cyclizine = Marezine[R]
Dorbanex = Danthron + poloxalkol = Dorbane[R]
  (Laxative)
Empronium Bromide = A parasympatholytic similar to atropine
Hexamine Hippurate = Methenamine Hippurate = Hiprex[R]
Hibitane = Chlorhexidine = Not available
Hyocine = Scopolamine
Ibuprofen = Motrin[R]
Indomethacin = Indocin[R]
Largactil = Chlorpromazine = Thorazine[R]
Linctus Methadone = Not available
Methotrimeprazine = Levoprome[R]
Metoclopramide = Not available
                (Antiemetic)
Milpar = Not available
                6% $Mg(OH)_2$ + 25% liquid paraffin
Nitrazepam = Not available
                (A benzodiazepine, Valium[R] class)
Noxyflex = Noxythiolin + Amethocaine = Not available
                (Antiseptic for irrigation of body cavities and fistulas)
Oxycodone Pectinate = Not available; however, oxycodone HC1
                is found in Percodan[R]
Pancrex V = Pancreatin = Viokase[R]
Paracetamol = Acetaminophen = Tylenol[R]
Phenazocine = A potent narcotic = Not available
Phenylbutazone = Butazolidine[R]
Polybactrin = spray Neomycin 495,000 u
                    Bacitracin 37,500 u
                    Polymixin B 150,000 m
Promazine = Sparine[R]

Salbutamol = Not available
Septrin = Trimethoprim/Sulfamethoxazole = Septra[R] or Bac-
   trim[R]
Stemetil = Prochlorperazine = Compazine[R]
Thioridazine = Mellaril[R]
Trimiprimine = Not available
      (A tricyclic antidepressant)

Pain-Comfort Chart: Hospice of Marin

APPENDIX C

Solid line: patient's perception of pain-comfort (10-1)
Broken line: dosage of Hospice Mix
Comfort attained for typical Hospice of Marin patient
(Chart prepared by W. M. Lamers, Jr. M.D., Medical Director, Hospice of Marin)

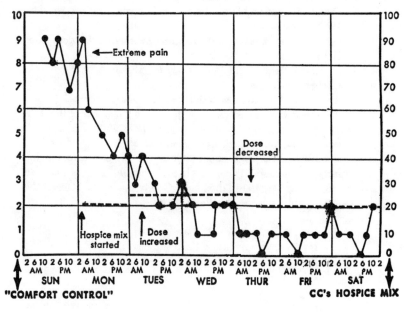

Notes

Chapter 1

1 The petition of the citizens of London is cited by Mary Rotha Clay in *The Medieval Hospital of England,* New York: Barnes & Noble, 1966, p. 236.

2 I am indebted throughout this work to Henri Nouwen for his development of the concept of *hospitality* in *The Wounded Healer,* New York: Doubleday, 1972, and, at greater length, in *Reaching Out,* New York: Doubleday, 1975.

3 Military terminology, interestingly enough, appears quite frequently in modern medical thought; e.g. "The Magic Bullet," "The War On Cancer," etc.

5 (Thomas) *The Lives of a Cell,* New York: Viking, 1974, p. 98.

6 *Dying,* directed and filmed by Michael Roemer, was produced by Michael Ambrosino.

   (Aries) *Western Attitudes Toward Death,* Baltimore: Johns Hopkins Press, 1974, p. 57.

8 (Reisman) *The Story of Medicine in the Middle Ages,* New York: Hoeber, 1935, p. 1.

   Agen hine: literally, *again servant.* Anglo-Saxon law stated that the visitor was a guest for three days, then a member of the staff. Three days was the traditional period of hospitality, after which the relationship was apt to change; and ancient proverbs reflect an ambivalent attitude about the host-guest relationship, ranging from the Chinese, "The host is happy when the guest is gone," to the Czech, "A guest in the house: God in the house." One of the most charming is the old Welsh rhyme:

   > Hail, guest, we ask not what thou art;
   > If friend, we greet thee, hand and heart;
   > If stranger, such no longer be;
   > If foe, our love shall conquer thee.

9 These statutes for care of the sick appear in *Medical Work of the Knights Hospitallers of St. John of Jerusalem,* edited by Edgar Erskine Hume, Baltimore: Johns Hopkins Press, 1940, pp. 28, 29.

10 (Saunders) "And From Sudden Death . . ." *Frontier,* Winter, 1961 (reprint), pp. 3, 5. Marya Mannes, so often a prophet in advance of contemporary thought, was one of the first American writers to discover the existence of the modern hospice in England; see her work, *Last Rights,* New York: Wm. Morrow, 1972.

Chapter 2

12 Dieter Jetter is quoted a number of times by John D. Thompson and Grace Goldin in their comprehensive and handsomely illustrated work, *The Hospital: A Social and Architectural History,* New Haven: Yale University Press, 1975, and it is regrettable that more of Jetter's work has not been translated into English; the passage quoted here appears in Thompson and Goldin, pp. 34-35. The quotation from Tolstoy is from "The Death of Ivan Ilych" in *The Death of Ivan Ilych and Other Stories,* New York: New American Library, 1960, p. 97. The plea of the patient entering a London hospice is recalled by Dr. Cicely Saunders.

Drawings and models of early Greek *Asklepieia* and Roman *valetudinaria* appear in Thompson and Goldin; medical procedure is described by Reisman, *op. cit.,* and by Mary Risley in *House of Healing,* New York: Doubleday, 1961. My own visit to the site of Epidaurus, when all the village talk was of Maria Callas, was in 1971.

18 Dr. Martin D. Netsky's moving article about the death of his mother appears in PHAROS, April, 1976, pp. 57-62.

21 (Emperor Julian) Cited in Risley, *House of Healing,* p. 93.

22 (Liegner) "St. Christopher's Hospice, 1974," *JAMA* 234:10, Dec. 8, 1975, p. 1048. Dr. Liegner, a specialist in Radiation Therapy, is a member of the Hospice Pilot Project team at St. Luke's Hospital in New York City.

(Rabbi Moses ben Maimon, also known as Maimonides) quoted in the *Bulletin of the Institute of the History of Medicine,* 3:585, 1935; cited in *Familiar Medical Quotations,* ed. Maurice B. Strauss, Boston: Little, Brown, 1968.

(Lois Wheeler Snow) *A Death With Dignity: When the Chinese Came,* New York: Random House, 1974, pp. 95, 104.

Chapter 3

24 (Pirsig) p. 13.
    (Clay) p. 207.
    (Nouwen) *Reaching Out,* p. 65.
28 The prayer, cited by Hume, *op. cit,* p. 111 (quoting Leon le
    Grand, "La Prière des Malades dans les Hôpitaux de St. Jean,"
    Paris, 1896) begins:

> Seigneurs Malades, pries pour pais que Dieu la mande de ciel
> en terre,
> Seigneurs Malades, pries pour le Fruit de la Terre que Dieu
> le multiple en tell maniere que saincte eglise en soit servie
> et le peuple soustanu,
> Seigneurs Malades, pries pour l'apostell de Rome et pour les
> Cardennaus et pour les patriarches et pour les archeves-
> ques et pour les evesques et les prelats . . .

Since our habits of speech are a powerful influence on our
behavior, it is interesting to imagine what subtle changes might
take place in a modern hospital if staff should refer to patients as
"My Lords" (using the same word generally used to refer to the
Supreme Being) and implored their aid daily in matters considered to be of crucial importance.

29 Hume (pp 50, 56) says that the incurably ill were set apart for the
    first time at Rhodes and that the eleven gallery rooms were
    evidently used for those in isolation and for pilgrims.
31 Descriptions and illustrations of early English hospices are to be
    found in Clay, *op. cit.* The price of a swan on the market in
    London in 1338 and other fascinating glimpses of medieval life
    are to be found in abundance in *The Knights Hospitallers in
    England: Being the Report of Prior Philip de Thame to the Grand
    Master Elyan de Villanova for AD 1338,* edited by Lambert B.
    Larking, New York: AMS Press, 1968.
34 (Brother Roger) "Frontiers of Pharmacology: The Middle Ages,"
    MD Magazine, August, 1976, p. 92.
36 (Beaune) Founded by a wealthy benefactor in 1443, the Hotel-
    Dieu at Beaune has the charm of a nobleman's country villa, with
    turrets and balconies facing into a central garden-court. Its "Hall
    of the Sick" with carved, vaulted roof over gracefully curtained

cubicles and a stained-glass window above the altar at the far end is perhaps the most beautiful room ever designed for medical care; and because of the quality of the art as well as the architecture, this place of healing has become a much-admired museum. For detailed description and illustrations, see *Les Villes d'Art Célèbres: Bordeaux, Dijon, Beaune,* by Charles Saunier, Paris: Libraire Renouard, 1925, pp. 146-54.

Chapter 4

37 (Phillips) p. 1.
40 "Private philanthropy has become the key supporter of city-sponsored out-of-hospital medical-care programs," writes Robert J. Blendon in "The Changing Role of Private Philanthropy in Health Affairs," *New England Journal of Medicine,* May 1, 1975. Private conscience and individual initiative, evidently, are the forces most likely to lead us out of the present morass. Meantime, it is rather mind-boggling to contemplate the superstructures of medical economics in comparison with the procedure of Hospitaller Knights in ancient Jerusalem: "It is the custom in this palace or hospital that every pilgrim should pay two Venetian pennies for the use of the hospital. If he sojourn there for a year he pays no more, if he abide but one day he pays no less" *Palestine Pilgrim's Text. Soc.,* Vol. XII, pp. 106-7, cited in Hume, p. 17.
52 Development of Hospice of Marin since the writing of Chapter 4 in November, 1976, can now be reported (July, 1977): The number of patient-family units now being cared for is regularly 22-23 per week, referred mainly by local physicians, and several physicians by now have become hospice patients themselves. Referrals now tend to come earlier in the illness, as the community has come to understand that the hospice is not only for help at the time of dying, but for help with living as fully as possible until death comes. Between October, 1976, and June, 1977, donations have been received from grateful friends and families of patients. Grants over a three-year period totaling $221,000 have been received from the S. H. Cowell Foundation, the San Francisco Foundation and the Vanguard Foundation, all of San Francisco; from St. Stephen's Church of Belvedere, California, from the Laras Foundation of Corte Madera, California, from the United Airlines Employees' Community Fund; and

from the Macomber Memorial Legacy, American Cancer Society. A full-fledged Bereavement Program is now in operation. Trained speakers are available to the community from the Speakers' Bureau of the hospice. "Friends of Hospice" numbering about forty are participating in many duties and functions. The administrative and patient-care staff now numbers twenty-three, with eleven experienced volunteers on hand. Regular staff still volunteer to a large extent, only six having token or part-time salaries. In October, 1977, Hospice of Marin will begin charging for those services which are reimbursable. Liability insurance for Board members had been arranged previously, but early in 1977, malpractice insurance as well was authorized for all those directly involved in patient-care. A "How-To of Hospice Care" conference in May, 1977 was jointly sponsored by Hospice of Marin, Hospice, Inc. of New Haven, Connecticut, and the Palliative Care Service of the Royal Victoria Hospital in Montreal. This conference, held at Dominican College in Marin County, California, was well-attended by visitors from seventeen states, including a large number of health-care professionals. In August, 1977, Dr. Cicely Saunders attended staff meetings at Hospice of Marin and gave a number of lectures on hospice care in the San Francisco area; in Fresno, California at St. Agnes Medical Center; and in Sacramento met with Governor Brown, Health Department personnel and legislators to discuss methods and standards of hospice care.

Chapter 5

53 (Risley) *op. cit.*, p. 166.
54 The young mother's case was reported in *The New York Tribune*, April 25, 1860 (cited by Gert H. Brieger, ed. *Medical America in the Nineteenth Century*, Baltimore: Johns Hopkins Press, 1972, p. 234).
56 (Public opinion) H. J. C. Gibson, quoted in George Rosen, *From Medical Police to Social Medicine*, New York: Science History Publications, 1974, p. 11.
58 Two sources of detailed information about nineteenth century workhouse conditions are, Risley's *House of Healing* and *The Hospitals, 1800-1948* by Brian Abel-Smith, London: Heinemann, 1964. Both quote the work of reformers who made on-site

investigations and reports at the time, horrified to discover situations where people not only starved and suffered untold physical miseries, but were treated with utmost contempt. It was not unusual, in such places, to find inmates forced to wash in their own urine, denied the simple amenities of fresh water, soap and lavatory paper simply because they were not considered to be truly human.

61 The statute against vagabondage is quoted at greater leangth by Risley, pp. 158-59, and includes the directive that "all persons are empowered to take idle children from vagabonds and retain them as apprentices until the boys become twenty-four years of age, and the girls twenty years; if they run away before the end of their apprenticeship, the masters can recover them, punish them with chains, and enslave them again. ... Masters are authorized to put a ring of iron around the neck, arm, or leg of their slaves ... for a surety of keeping them." This law, impossible to enforce, was shortly thereafter rescinded; and in any case should not be taken to represent the policy of Edward VI, who was very young at the time and caught in a power struggle between ambitious advisors, large landowners, and chiefs of state.

62 (Humanitarianism of the successful) *A History of Public Health*, New York: MD Publications, 1958, p. 137. The humanitarianism of the successful is also likely to be tempered by their realization that, if the helpless cannot be held accountable for their condition, then no moral superiority accrues to those who have climbed above.

("Uneconomic aberrations") John Langdon-Davies, *Westminster Hospital*, London: John Murray, 1952, p. 16.

(Selection of patients for teaching and research) Abel-Smith, *op. cit.*, p. 46.

65 (Nightingale) From *Notes on Hospitals*, cited by Risley, p. 193. George Pickering's delightful book, *Creative Malady*, New York: Dell, 1974, gives a detailed account of Florence Nightingale's psychosomatic ailments, taking the view that they gave her the privacy and freedom she needed for her creative work.

Chapter 6

69 (Holden) "Hospices For the Dying: Relief From Pain and Fear," *Science*, July 30, 1976, p. 390.

(Phillips) "St. Christopher's Hospice: Annual Report, 1975-6," p. 36.
It should be noted that quite near the spacious lawns and gardens of St. Christopher's immediate neighborhood, there are crowded areas far less affluent; residents here are considered to be very much a part of the hospice community, too.

80   In May, 1977, after a series of comparative pharmacological studies, morphine in suitably large amounts was substituted for diamorphine in the St. Christopher's Hospice Mix, without any difficulty noted. For further information on this question, see R. G. Twycross, "Choice of Strong Analgesic in Terminal Cancer: Diamorphine or Morphine?" in *Pain*, The Journal of the International Study of Pain, 3:2, April, 1977, pp. 93-104.

Chapter 7

100   The patient described here as "Mrs. Kent" was, at the time I met her, far closer to death than I (or perhaps she) realized. After being discharged once again from St. Christopher's she went to stay with a close friend, who wrote me, "Mrs. —— has now returned home, which is what she and her 'extended family' always wanted. The lounge in my house has been turned into her bedroom. The hatch to the kitchen is permanently open and even in her now very drowsy state she hears, and warms to, the familiar noises of our daily routine. And the care, the all-enveloping and strengthening care, given by St. Christopher's Out-patients' service, continues ..." And later, "She died peacefully and surrounded by both her own and my family, on the evening of January 31st, 1977."

104   The experience of the woman known here as Lillian Preston is reminiscent of the writings of an ancient Venetian, Louis Coronaro (1464-1566) who reported at the age of 95: "At this extreme age of mine, I enjoy two lives at the same time: one, the earthly, which I possess in reality; the other, the heavenly, which I possess in thought.... And I hold that our departure from this world is not death, but merely a passage which the soul makes from this earthly life to the heavenly one, immortal and infinitely perfect." *The Art of Living Long*, Milwaukee: William F. Butler, 1903, pp. 110-111.

Chapter 8

107 (Fletcher) "The Patient's Right to Die," *Harpers,* 221:1325, October, 1960, p. 141.

111 (Eliot) "Little Gidding" from "Four Quartets" in *The Complete Poems and Plays,* New York: Harcourt, Brace and World, 1934, p. 139.

118 The senselessness of pain in incurable disease is a subject discussed by many writers on modern hospice care: see works by Saunders, Twycross, Lamerton and others in Bibliography; also, L. LeShan, "The World of the Patient in Severe Pain of Long Duration," *Journal of Chronic Diseases,* 1964:17, pp. 119-126.
(Dickinson) in *Final Harvest: ED's Poems,* edited by T. H. Johnson, Boston: Little, Brown, 1961.

Chapter 9

123 (Belloc) *The Cruise of the Nona,* Boston: Houghton Mifflin, 1925, p. 161.

124 Quotations from Jonathan Edwards in this chapter are from his "Images or Shadows of Divine Things" (edited by Perry Miller) in *Colonial American Writing,* second edition, edited by Roy Harvey Pearce, New York: Holt, Rinehart & Winston, 1969, pp. 370-75.

126 (Wishes of cancer patients) "Terminal Care: Issues and Alternatives," Claire F. Ryder and Diane M. Ross, *Public Health Reports,* Jan/Feb 1977, states that 67% of the patients surveyed expressed the desire to die at home as opposed to the 20% who were able to do so. The two groups most successful in achieving their wishes in this respect were (1), upper-income people, on account of their ability to hire suitable caretakers with private funds and (2), the low socioeconomic group on account of Medicaid and support supplied by cohesive family units. It was the middle class, middle-income people who suffered most from the present system. Ryder and Ross also cite a study by Cancer Care, Inc., in 1973, showing the median cost of dying of cancer as $19,055, two and two-thirds times more than the median family income that year of $8,000. Hospice care, of course, extends itself to persons of all social and economic groups, but can obviously offer a service badly needed by those "caught in the middle."

129 (Carter's campaign speeches) Quoted in "The Health Cost 'Crisis,' " *Medical World News*, Feb. 21, 1977, pp. 57-72.

156 (The young musician) Hospice, Inc. staff arranged shortly after my visit to contact this patient's father, who came from out of state—though in poor health at the time himself—to see his son for the first time in 14 years. At this meeting, the two were reconciled. Then, on August 23, 1977, I received a call from the hospice letting me know that the patient was near death. Among his last words were a request that I should use his real name in this book. I telephoned him and promised him, just before he died, that I would. *Fare well, Jim Burnham.*

Chapter 10

157 (Tennyson) *Idylls of the King,* New York: Airmont, 1969, p. 251.

158 (Wigglesworth) Cited by John B. Blake in *Public Health In the Town of Boston, 1630-1822,* Cambridge: Harvard University Press, 1959, p. 4.

159 Mention of the arrest and deportation of a Widow Paige and her family at this time appears in John B. Blake, *ibid.*

160 Benjamin Franklin's delight in his methods of raising funds for the founding of Philadelphia General Hospital is described and documented by Thompson and Goldin, *op. cit.,* p. 97.

161 ("A Cup of cold water . . .") From *The Papers of Benjamin Franklin,* cited by Thompson and Goldin, p. 97.
     (Physicians' income) "On The Other Hand," by Uwe E. Reinhardt, *Medical World News,* Feb. 21, 1977, p. 108.

164 On the corporate power of hospitals at the turn of the century, see "The Use and Abuse of Medical Charities in Late Nineteenth Century America," by Gert H. Brieger, *American Journal of Public Health,* March, 1977, 67:3, pp. 264-67.

167 Some abuses of the hospice concept may be expected merely as a result of normal bureaucratic chaos with its accompanying habits of exploitation and petty pilferage: "As soon as the government gets an idea that is useful, helpful, and in the best health interests of the country, instantly suppliers of goods of services perceive it as a pot of gold, knowing that no effective controls will be applied" (Sidney Wolfe, chief of Ralph Nader's Health Research group, *San Francisco Examiner,* August 29, 1976).
     Others, however, may be far more sinister. During 1976, a "non-

profit organization" headquartered in Fort Lauderdale, Florida, sought funds for something called "The Heavenly Rest" which they identified as a "hospice to be located in Central America similar to the St. Christopher's Hospice in London, run by Cicely Saunders." Under their regime, supported, they claim, by an individual "who represents strong Latin-American interests," terminally ill patients would have been shipped to Central America, lectured for three days about the beauties of the afterlife, then given poison and cremated, "the package price for the total job" being "less than $1,000 where the travel distance does not exceed 1800 miles." The implication that such a loathsome plan resembles in any way the work of Dr. Saunders— or the work of any legitimate hospice here or abroad—is slanderous as well as patently absurd. National legislation on standards of hospice care, and on the use of the name "hospice" may well be necessary in order to protect the public interest, and the integrity of the hospice concept, against such misguided and/ or deliberately deceitful entrepreneurs as this.

Chapter 11

172   ("Getting to Know St. Joseph's Hospice,") (pamphlet), London: St. Joseph's Hospice, p. 9.

("He drew a circle ...) Barbara Hill, Executive Director of Hospice of Marin, uses this version of the poem by Edwin Markham when speaking before various groups about the hospice concept. The original poem, "Outwitted," appears in *Magic Ring: A Collection of Verse*, edited by Ruth A. Brown, Bridgeport: Seven Seas Press, 1937, p. 62.

181   A letter from Balfour M. Mount, M.D., August 8, 1977, expresses disagreement with my opinion that "much here is missing" in the community life of the PCS. "Not only has there been a christening," he writes, "and visits from bridal parties, complete with flowing gowns and confetti, but the regular celebration of birthdays, the visiting of children and pets (including, on one occasion, a part timber wolf) but the regular celebration of life and its small details, the playing poker for penny chips with volunteers while sipping a good scotch, singsongs with patients and staff."

183   (Twycross, "Ten Commandments") From "Principles and Prac-

tice of the Relief of Pain in Terminal Cancer," (reprint) *Update*, July, 1972.

184 In connection with Sir Michael Sobell House, it should be mentioned that, due in large part to the efforts of Major Garnett, Secretary to the National Society for Cancer Relief, a number of Continuing Care Units similar to this one are now opening in England. SMS House was the fourth of its type to open; previous Units were founded at Bournemouth, Southampton and Northampton.

189 In the United States, more than in Great Britain, the word "Home" is apt to have unfortunate connotations when used in connection with an institution or an inpatient facility. We have seen too many "Homes" which were scandalously inadequate places for the helpless or the elderly to be kept out of the main stream of life. In England, too, the word "homely" means home-like and cozy, whereas in the U.S.A. it means ugly and plain. Dr. Gusterson has chosen the word "Home" for the very reasons that might influence an American Medical Director to avoid it!

193 (Lamerton) From "Euthanasia" (reprint), *Nursing Times*, February 21, 1974.

194 (Lamerton) *Ibid.* Aside from the humanitarian service provided by St. Joseph's Domiciliary Care Service, the financial savings are noteworthy. In the year 1976, this team cared for 263 patients, 44.9 percent of them dying at home. The care of these patients would have cost the National Health Service (had they gone into hospitals such as St. Barts) no less than £63,000. But the total amount contributed to St. Joseph's for this service in 1976 by National Health was £20,000, and the expenditures for the Domiciliary Care Service were £11,843.03. The National Society for Cancer Relief and the NHS have joined a great variety of private and corporate donors to support the work of the hospice, as is typical in the case of most of these facilities, both in America and in the United Kingdom.

196 (Nouwen) p. 69.

Chapter 12

198 (Congreve) From the preface of *The Book of the Craft of Dying and Other Early English Tracts Concerning Death*, edited by Frances M.M. Comper, New York: Arno Press, 1977, p. xxxv.

Spenser's *The Faerie Queene* (1:X:xxxvi) shows the troubled hero taking refuge in a traditional hospice setting:

> Eftsoones unto a holy hospitall,
> That was foreby the way, she did him bring;
> In which seven Bead-men, that had vowed all
> Their life to service of high heaven's King,
> Did spend their daies in doing godly thing.
> Their gates to all were open evermore,
> That by the wearie way were travelling;
> And one sate wayting ever them before,
> To call in commers-by that needy were and poore.

200 (Juiraros) Robert W. Habenstein and William M. Lamers, *Funeral Customs The World Over*, Milwaukee: Bulfin, 1963, p. 22. For information about death customs of Navajo, Mexican, African and many of the Asian groups mentioned in this chapter, I am indebted to this work.

201 (Solzhenitsyn) *The Cancer Ward*, New York: Dial Press, 1968, p. 97.

(Byrne) *Destiny Bay*, Boston: Little, Brown, 1928, p. 28.

203 (Bonhoeffer) cited by M.C. McCoy in *To Die With Style!*, New York: Abingdon Press, 1974, p. 112.

204 (Eliot) *Op. cit.*, pp. 144, 145.

206 (Moody subjects) pp. 48, 49.

207 (Kübler-Ross) p. 136.

A patient of Dr. Cicely Saunders, after telling of a "near death experience," then reported, "Quite recently I have been ill again, and then I did think at one time that I was going back to where I had been before. I seemed to know where I was, and I can remember thinking suddenly, 'I've got something to do, I must arrange my elder son's Bar Mitzvah, nobody else *could* do it as my husband is not Jewish, and I dreamt—I'm sure it was a dream—that I said 'If it's all the same to you Lord, I can't go just yet, I've got something to do' and I seemed to hear in my dream a laughing voice saying, 'Well, if you think you are the only one who can do it, stay,' And then in the dream I heard the most beautiful voice—I've never heard a voice like it, nothing in my life—saying 'I wouldn't have you come to Me fretting.'" (Private correspondence, used by permission.)

208 (Death as a journey) Carl Jung writes: "In my rather long
     psychological experience I have observed a great many people
     whose unconscious psychic activity I was able to follow into the
     immediate presence of death. As a rule, the approaching end was
     indicated by those symbols which, in normal life also, proclaim
     changes of psychological condition—rebirth symbols such as
     changes of locality, journeys, and the like." (In "The Soul and
     Death," from *The Meaning of Death,* edited by Herman Feifel,
     New York: McGraw-Hill, 1969, p. 10). In a near-death experience
     of his own, reported in *Memories, Dreams, Reflections,* New York:
     Random House, 1965, pp. 289-97, Dr. Jung felt freed of the "box-
     system" of three-dimensional existence and entered a realm of
     spiritual ecstasy, "a non-temporal state in which present, past and
     future are one." His nurse told him afterward, "It was as if you
     were surrounded by a bright glow" and, "that was a phenomenon
     she had sometimes observed in the dying, she added."
209 *(Ars Moriendi)* pp. 93, 36.
210 (Jacob) *Science,* 196:4295, June 10, 1977, p. 1166.
     ("Go, go, go, said the bird." T.S. Eliot, "Burnt Norton," *op cit.,* p.
     118.)
212 ("Dying is the experience of a lifetime") These were the last
     words of Marian Murdock Rattray, Marin County, California,
     September 5, 1976.
     For development of my thoughts on personal growth throughout
     this book I am indebted to George B. Leonard's illuminating
     work, *The Transformation,* New York: Delacorte Press, 1972.

Bibliography

Asterisk * indicates item giving information about modern hospice concept and/or procedure.

Abel-Smith, Brian. *The Hospice: 1800-1948*. London: Heinemann, 1964.

Addis, Thomas. *Glomerular Nephritis, Diagnosis and Treatment*. New York: Macmillan, 1948.

Alsofrom, Judy. "The Hospice Way of Dying," *American Medical News* (Feb. 21, 1977), pp. 7-9. *

Alsop, Stewart. *Stay of Execution*. Philadelphia: Lippincott, 1973.

Aries, Philippe. *Western Attitudes Toward Death From the Middle Ages to the Present*. Baltimore: Johns Hopkins Press, 1974.

Aring, Charles. *The Understanding Physician*. Detroit: Wayne University Press, 1971.

Ashley, Beth. "Death Without Pain: A Dying Man Tells How Hospice Helps" (reprint), *Independent-Journal*, San Rafael, California, Nov. 15, 1976. *

Baker, Canon John Austin. "Why Should This Happen To Me?" Text of an address given at St. Christopher's Hospice, London, October 20, 1975. *

Banashek, Susan. "Family—The Best Medicine," *San Francisco Chronicle*, May 11, 1976, p. 17. *

Baqui, Mufti Abdul and Rabbi B. Joseph. "Jewish and Muslim Teaching Concerning Death: A St. Joseph's Hospice Occasional Paper." London: St. Joseph Hospice.

Barber, Bernard. "Compassion in Medicine: Toward New Definitions and New Institutions," *New England Journal of Medicine*, 295:7 (Oct. 21, 1976), pp. 939-43.

Barnard, C. N. "Good Death at St. Christopher's Hospice," *Family Health*, 5:40ff, April, 1973. *

Bartlett, Linda and Bryan Hodgson. "Love, the Final Act of Life," *Washington Post*, April 24, 1977. *

Becker, Earnest. *The Denial of Death*. New York: Free Press, 1973.

Belloc, Hilaire. *The Cruise of the Nona.* Boston: Houghton Mifflin, 1925.

Bettman, Otto L. *A Pictorial History of Medicine.* Springfield: Charles C Thomas, 1956.

Blake, John B. *Public Health in the Town of Boston, 1630-1822.* Cambridge: Harvard University Press, 1959.

Blendon, Robert J. "The Changing Role of Private Philanthropy in Health Affairs," *New England Journal of Medicine,* 295:7 (August 12, 1976), pp. 367-9.

Braunfels, Wolfgang. *Monasteries of Western Europe.* Princeton: Princeton University Press, 1973.

Brieger, Gert H. ed. *Medical America in the Nineteenth Century.* Baltimore: Johns Hopkins Press, 1972.

——, "The Use and Abuse of Medical Charities in Late Nineteenth Century America," *American Journal of Public Health,* 67:3 (March, 1977), pp. 264-7.

Brooke, Christopher. *Medieval Church and Society.* London: Sidgwick and Jackson, 1971.

Brown, Norman O. *Life Against Death.* Middletown: Wesleyan University Press, 1959.

Brown, Ruth A., ed. *Magic Ring: A Collection of Verse.* Rev. ed. Bridgeport: Seven Seas Press, 1937.

Buber, Martin. *I And Thou.* New York: Scribner, 1970.

Buckingham, Robert, Joan Kron and Henry Wald. *The Hospice Concept.* New York Health Sciences Pub. Corp., 1977. °

Budge, E. A. Wallis, ed. *The Book of the Dead.* London: Kegan Paul, Trench, Trübner, 1909.

Bunyan, John. *The Pilgrim's Progress.* New York: Scribner, 1918.

Byrne, Donn. *Destiny Bay.* Boston: Little, Brown, 1928.

Chan, Lo-Yi. "Hospice: A New Building Type to Comfort the Dying," (reprint) *AIA Journal,* Dec., 1976. °

Charles, Eleanor. "A Hospice for the Terminally Ill," *New York Times,* March 13, 1977. °

Choron, Jacques. *Death and Western Thought.* New York: Collier, 1963.

Church, Richard. *Portrait of Canterbury.* London: Hutchinson, 1968.

Clay, Mary Rotha. *The Medieval Hospital of England.* New York: Barnes and Noble, 1966.

Colen, B. D. "Nurse's Speciality: Care for the Dying," *Washington Post* (August 24, 1975), pp A1-4. °

Comper, Frances M. M., ed. *The Book of the Craft of Dying and Other Early English Tracts Concerning Death.* New York: Arno Press, 1977.

Cornaro, Louis. *The Art of Living Long.* Milwaukee: William F. Butler, 1903.

Cousins, Norman. "Anatomy of an Illness (As Perceived by the Patient)," *New England Journal of Medicine,* 295:26 (Dec. 23, 1976), pp. 1458-1463.

Craven, Joan and Florence S. Wald. "Hospice Care for Dying Patients," *American Journal of Nursing,* 75:10 (Oct., 1975), pp. 1816-22. °

Crowther, Bishop C. Edward. "Care V. Cure in the Treatment of the Terminally Ill," Report, Center for the Study of Democratic Institutions, April, 1976, pp 20-23. °

DeFouw, Ruth. "Hospices for the Dying," *The Humanist,* July/August, 1974, pp 28-9. °

Dempsey, David. *The Way We Die: An Investigation of Death in America Today.* New York: Macmillan, 1975.

Dickinson, Emily. *Final Harvest: ED's Poems,* ed. T. H. Johnson. Boston: Little, Brown, 1961.

Dobihal, Edward F. "Talk or Terminal Care?" *Connecticut Medicine,* 38:7 (July, 1974), pp. 364-67. °

———, S. Lack, D. Rezendes, F. Wald. "Principles of Hospice Care." (2/19/75). New Haven: Hospice, Inc. °

Downie, P. A. "Havens of Peace: Hostels for Terminal Patients," *Nursing Times,* 69:1068-70 (August 16, 1973). °

Downing, A. B., ed. *Euthanasia and the Right to Death.* London: Owen, 1969.

Dunphy, J. Englebert. "On Caring for the Patient With Cancer," *New England Journal of Medicine,* 295:6 (August 5, 1976), pp. 313-19. °

Eggleston, Edward. *The Transit of Civilization From England to America in the Seventeenth Century.* Boston: Beacon Press, 1959.

Eissler, Kurt Robert. *The Psychiatrist and the Dying Patient.* New York: International Universities Press, 1955.

Eliot, T. S. *The Complete Poems and Plays.* New York: Harcourt, Brace and World, 1934.

Elliott, Sumner Locke. *Going.* New York: Harper and Row, 1975.

Erikson, Joan. *Activity, Recovery, Growth.* New York: Norton, 1976.

Evans-Wentz, W. Y., ed. *The Tibetan Book of the Dead.* London: Oxford University Press, 1960.

Feifel, Herman, ed. *The Meaning of Death.* New York: McGraw-Hill, 1969.

Field, Minna. *Patients Are People: A Medical-Social Approach to Prolonged Illness.* New York: Columbia University Press, 1967.

"Filling the Gap Between Home and Hospital: St. Ann's Hospice, England," *Nursing Mirror*, 134:17 (Feb. 4, 1972). °

Fletcher, J. F. "The Patient's Right to Die," *Harpers*, 221:1325 (Oct., 1960), pp. 138-43.

Formby, Fr. John, Rev. Michael Hickey and Rev. Gordon Jones. "Christian Teaching Concerning Death: A St. Joseph's Hospice Occasional Paper." London: St. Joseph's Hospice.

"For the Terminally Ill, A Hospital That Cares: St. Christopher's Hospice, London," *Medical World News*, 15:46-7 (July 19, 1974).°

Foss, Martin. *Death, Sacrifice and Tragedy*. Lincoln: University of Nebraska Press, 1966.

Frankl, Viktor E. *Man's Search For Meaning: An Introduction to Logotherapy*. Boston: Beacon Press, 1959.

Freud, Sigmund. *Civilization, War and Death*, ed. John Richman. London: Hogarth Press, 1953.

Friedenwald, Harry. "The Ethics of the Practice of Medicine From the Jewish Point of View," *Johns Hopkins Hospital Bulletin* 318:256-61 (August, 1917).

"Frontiers of Pharmacology: The Middle Ages," *MD Magazine*, August 1976, pp 83-95.

Fulton, Robert. *Death and Identity*. New York: John Wiley, 1945.

Garner, Jim. "Palliative Care: It's the Quality of Life Remaining That Matters," *CMA Journal*, 115:179-80 (July 17, 1976). °

"Getting To Know St. Joseph's Hospice," (pamphlet). London: St. Joseph's Hospice. °

Gimpel, Jean. *The Medieval Machine*. New York: Holt, Rinehart, Winston, 1976.

Glaser, Barney G. and Anselm L. Strauss. *Awareness of Dying*. Chicago: Aldine, 1965.

Goleman, Daniel. "We are Breaking the Silence About Death," *Psychology Today*, Sept., 1976, p. 44f. °

Gorer, Geoffrey. *Death, Grief and Mourning*. New York: Doubleday, 1965.

Habenstein, Robert W. and William M. Lamers. *Funeral Customs the World Over*. Milwaukee: Bulfin, 1963.

——, *The History of American Funeral Directing*. Milwaukee: Bulfin, 1955.

Hendin, David. *Death As A Fact of Life*. New York: Norton, 1973.°

Hines, William. "An Easier Way of Death for Victims of Cancer," *Chicago Sun-Times*, August 29, 1975, p. B7°

Holden, Constance. "Hospices for the Dying: Relief From Pain and Fear," *Science* (July 30, 1976), pp. 389-91. °

"Home Care of the Cancer Patient," *Proceedings*, American Cancer Society Conference, May 10, 1973. Syracuse, N.Y.

"Hospice For The Dying Planned in Greater New Haven," *Hospital Management*, 112:19 (August, 1973). °

"Hospice: Pilot Project," (pamphlet). New York: St. Luke's Hospital Center. °

"Hospice," *Thanatos* (March, 1977), pp. 6-11. °

Hume, Edgar Erskine. *Medical Work of the Knights Hospitallers of St. John of Jerusalem*. Baltimore: Johns Hopkins Press, 1940.

Illich, Ivan. *Medical Nemesis*. New York: Random House, 1976.

Imbert, Jean. *Les Hôpitaux en France*. Paris: Presses Univ., 1958.

Ingles, Thelma. "St. Christopher's Hospice," *Nursing Outlook*, 22:12 (Dec., 1974), pp. 759-63. °

Jacob, François. "Evolution and Tinkering," *Science*, 196:4295 (June 10, 1977), pp. 1161-66.

James, William. *The Varieties of Religious Experience*. New York: Longmans Green, 1902.

Jordan, Lynette. "Hospice in America," *The Coevolution Quarterly* (Summer, 1977), pp. 112-15. °

Joy, Charles R., ed. *Albert Schweitzer: An Anthology*. Boston: Beacon Press, 1947.

Jung, C. G. *Memories, Dreams, Reflections*. New York: Random House, 1965.

Kastenbaum, R. "Toward Standards of Care for the Terminally Ill: That A Need Exists," *Omega*, 6:2 (1975); p. 77.

Keleman, Stanley. *Living Your Dying*. New York: Random House, 1974.

Kerppola-Sirola, Irma. "The Death of an Old Professor," *JAMA*, 232:7 (May 19, 1975), pp. 728-9.

Kerstein, M. D. "Care For the Terminally Ill: A Hospice," *American Journal of Psychiatry* 129:237-38 (August, 1972). °

Kilduff, Marshall. "Another Way To Treat The Dying," *San Francisco Chronicle*, April 10, 1975, p. 43. °

Krant, M. J. *Dying and Dignity: The Meaning and Control of a Personal Death*. Springfield: Charles C. Thomas, 1974.

Kron, Joan. "Designing A Better Place To Die," *New York Magazine*, March 1, 1976, pp. 43-49. °

———, "Learning To Live With Death," *Philadelphia Magazine*, April, 1973, p. 82f.

——, "The Good News About the Bad News," *New York Magazine,* July 21, 1975. °

Kübler-Ross, Elisabeth. *Death, The Final Stage of Growth.* Englewood: Prentice-Hall, 1975. °

——, *On Death and Dying.* New York: Macmillan, 1969. °

——, *Questions and Answers on Death and Dying.* New York: Macmillan, 1974. °

Lack, Sylvia. "Philosophy and Organization of a Hospice Program," (pamphlet). New Haven: Hospice, Inc. °

Lamerton, Richard and Sylvia Lack, eds. *The Hour of Our Death.* London: Macmillan, 1974. °

Lamerton, Richard. "Euthanasia" (reprint) *Nursing Times,* Feb. 21, 1974. °

——, "The Need For Hospices," *Nursing Times,* 71:155-57 (Jan. 23, 1975). °

——, "Vegetables?" (reprint) *Nursing Times,* Aug. 1, 1974. °

Langdon-Davies, John. *Westminster Hospital.* London: John Murray, 1952.

Larking, Lambert B., ed. *The Knights Hospitallers in England: Being the Report of Prior Philip de Thame to the Grand Master Elyan de Villanova for AD 1338.* New York: AMS Press, 1968.

Leonard, George B. *The Transformation.* New York: Delacorte Press, 1972.

LeShan, L. "The World of the Patient in Severe Pain of Long Duration," *Journal of Chronic Diseases,* 1964:17, pp. 119-26. °

Lewis, C. S. *A Grief Observed.* New York: Seabury Press, 1961.

Lewis, Tony. "Hospice Gave Them An Alternative" (reprint) *Twin Cities Times,* Corte Madera, California, March 30, 1977.°

——, "Hospice of Marin: Caring for the Terminally Ill at Home" (reprint) *Twin Cities Times,* Corte Madera, California, March 30, 1977. °

Liegner, Leonard M. "St. Christopher's Hospice, 1974," *JAMA* 234:10 (Dec. 8, 1975), pp. 1047,48. °

Mannes, Marya. *Last Rights.* New York: Wm. Morrow, 1972. °

Marshall, Victor W. "Socialization for Impending Death in a Retirement Village," *American Journal of Sociology,* 80:5, pp. 1124-44.

May, Rollo. *Power And Innocence.* New York: Norton, 1972.

——, and Robert McCrie. "The Meaning of Anxiety," *Practical Psychology For Physicians* (May, 1976), pp. 46-52.

McCoy, Marjorie C. *To Die With Style!* New York: Abingdon Press, 1974.

McNulty, Barbara. "St. Christopher's Out-Patients," *American Journal of Nursing* (Dec., 1971), pp. 2328-30. °

——, "The Needs of the Dying." Text of a lecture given to the Guild of Pastoral Psychology, Jan., 1969, St. Christopher's Hospice, London.°

Miller, Perry. *Jonathan Edwards.* New York: Meridian Books, 1959.

Mitchell, Henry. "Of Death and Living: Finding Succor in a Time of Dread," *Washington Post,* May 25, 1975, p. F1.

Moody, Raymond A., Jr. *Life After Life.* Atlanta: Mockingbird Books, 1975.

Mount, Balfour M., Allan Jones and Andrew Patterson, "Death and Dying: Attitudes in a General Hospital," *Urology* IV:6 (Dec., 1974), pp. 741-47.

——, I. Ajemian and J. F. Scott, "Use of the Brompton Mixture in Treating the Chronic Pain of Malignant Disease," *CMA Journal,* July 17, 1976, pp. 122-28. °

——, "The Problems of Caring for the Dying in a General Hospital," *CMA Journal,* July 17, 1976, pp. 119-24. °

Neihardt, John G. *Black Elk Speaks.* New York: Pocketbooks, 1962.

Netsky, Martin D. "Dying in a System of 'Good Care': Case Report and Analysis." *PHAROS,* April, 1976, pp. 57-61.

"New Haven Hospice Provides Home Care for the Terminally Ill," (reprint) *American Journal of Nursing,* 74:717 (April, 1974). °

Nouwen, Henri. *Reaching Out.* New York: Doubleday, 1975.

——, *The Wounded Healer.* New York: Doubleday, 1972.

——, *With Open Hands.* Notre Dame: Ave Maria Press, 1972.

"On Dying At Home," *Emergency Medicine,* Feb., 1977, pp. 137-41.

"On Dying Well: An Anglican Contribution To The Debate on Euthanasia," (pamphlet). London: Yelf Bros., 1975.

"Optimum Care For Hopelessly Ill Patients," *New England Journal of Medicine,* 295:7 (August 12, 1976), pp. 362-4.

Osler, Sir William. *The Student Life and Other Essays.* Boston: Houghton Mifflin, 1931.

"Palliative Care Service: Pilot Project." Montreal: Royal Victoria Hospital, McGill University, 1976. °

Parkes, Colin Murray. *Bereavement: Studies of Grief in Adult Life.* Middlesex: Penguin, 1975.

——, "Components of the Reaction to Loss of a Limb, Spouse or Home," *Journal of Psychosomatic Research,* 16:343-49.

——, "Effects of Bereavement on Physical and Mental Health—A Study of the Medical Records of Widows," *British Medical Journal,* August 1, 1964, pp. 274-79.

——, "Grief As An Illness" (reprint) *New Society,* April 9, 1964.

——, "What Becomes of Redundant World Models? A Contribution to the Study of Adaptation to Change," *British Journal of Medical Psychology* (1975), 48:131-37.

Pearce, Roy Harvey, ed. *Colonial American Writing.* Second edition. New York: Holt, Rinehart and Winston, 1969.

Pellouchoud, Canoine Alfred. "Le Grand Saint-Bernard," (pamphlet). Lausanne: Hospice de St. Bernard, 1969.

Phillips, Michael. *The Seven Laws of Money.* New York: Random House, 1974.

Pickering, George. *Creative Malady.* New York: Dell, 1974.

Pirsig, R. M. *Zen and the Art of Motorcycle Maintenance.* New York: Bantam, 1974.

Powledge, Tabitha M. "Death As An Acceptable Subject," *New York Times,* July 25, 1976. IV:8 •

Quint, Jeanne. *The Nurse and the Dying Patient.* New York: Macmillan, 1967.

Rabkin, Mitchell J., Gerald Gillerman and Nancy Rice. "Orders Not To Resuscitate," *New England Journal of Medicine,* 295:7 (August 12, 1976), pp. 364-66.

Reinhardt, Uwe E. "On The Other Hand," *Medical World News,* Feb. 21, 1977, p. 108.

Reisman, David. *The Story of Medicine in the Middle Ages.* New York: Hoeber, 1935.

Renwick, E. D. *A Short History of the Order of St. John.* London: Swindon Press, 1958.

Rhein, Reginald W. Jr. "The Health Cost 'Crisis,' " *Medical World News,* Feb. 21, 1977, pp. 57-72.

Risley, Mary. *House of Healing.* New York: Doubleday, 1961.

Roach, Nancy. "The Last Day of April," (pamphlet). California Division, American Cancer Society, 1974.

Roberts, Janice and Walter Blum. "A Death In My Family," California Living Section, *San Francisco Chronicle,* April 21, 1974.

Rosen, George. *A History of Public Health.* New York: MD Publications, 1958.

——, *From Medical Police to Social Medicine.* New York: Science History Publications, 1974.

Rosenbaum, Ernest H. and Isadora R. *Mind and Body: A Rehabilitation*

Guide for Patients and their Families. San Francisco, 1977 (work in progress).

Rosenthal, Ted. *How Could I Not Be Among You?* New York: Braziller, 1973.

Rossman, Parker. "A Prophetic Ministry to the Dying," *The Christian Century* (April 21, 1976), pp. 384-87. °

Ryder, Claire F. and Diane M. Ross. "Terminal Care: Issues And Alternatives," *Public Health Reports* (Jan./Feb. 1977), pp. 20-29.°

Sackett, Walter W. Jr. "Death With Dignity," *Medical Opinion And Review* (June, 1969), pp. 25-31.

"St. Barnabas At Prayer," (pamphlet). Worthing, England: St. Barnabas' Home. °

"St. Christopher's Hospice: Annual Report" (pamphlets: 1973-4, 1974-5, 1975-6). London: St. Christopher's Hospice. °

Saunders, Cicely. "And From Sudden Death ..." (reprint) *Frontier,* Winter, 1961. °

———, "Care of The Dying," *A Nursing Times Publication* (second edition). London, 1976. °

———, *Care Of the Dying.* London: Macmillan, 1959. °

———, "Essentials For A Hospice" (privately printed by St. Christopher's Hospice, London, 1976.). °

———, "I Was Sick And You Visited Me," *In the Service of Medicine: A Quarterly Paper,* 42:2 (July, 1965).°

———, "Telling Patients" (reprint) *District Nursing,* Sept., 1965. °

———, "Terminal Care," in *Medical Oncology,* ed. K. D. Bagshawe. Oxford: Blackwell Scientific Publications, 1973. °

———, "The Challenge of Terminal Care," in *Scientific Foundations of Oncology,* ed. T. Symington and R. L. Carter. London: Heinemann, 1975. °

———, "The Last Stages of Life," *American Journal of Nursing* (March, 1965), pp. 70-75. °

———, "The Management of Fatal Illness in Childhood," *Proceedings of the Royal Society of Medicine,* 62:6 (June, 1969), pp. 550-53. °

———, "The Management of Terminal Illness," (reprint) *Hospital Publications, Ltd.* London, 1967. °

———, "The Nature and Management of Pain in Terminal Malignant Disease." Script of a tape for the Medical Recording Service (third edition). London, 1975. °

———, "The Need for Inpatient Care for the Patient With Terminal Cancer," *Middlesex Hospital Journal,* 72:3 (Feb., 1973). °

————, "The Need for Institutional Care for the Patient With Advanced Cancer," in *Anniversary Volume,* Cancer Institute, Madras, 1964.°

————, "The Symptomatic Treatment of Incurable Malignant Disease," *Prescriber's Journal* (Oct., 1964), pp. 68-73. °

————, "Training for the Practice of Clinical Gerontology: The Role of Social Medicine," *Interdisciplinary Topics of Gerontology,* 5:72-78, 1970.°

————, "Treatment of Intractable Pain in Terminal Cancer," *Proceedings of the Royal Society of Medicine,* 56:191. °

————, "Watch With Me" (reprint) *Nursing Times,* Nov. 26, 1965.°

————, ed. *The Management of Terminal Malignant Disease.* London: Edward Arnold (in press, 1977).

Saunier, Charles. *Les Villes d'Art Célèbres: Bordeaux, Dijon, Beaune,* ed. H. Laurens (deuxième edition). Paris: Libraire Renouard, 1925.

Schnack, Ingeborg. *Rilke in Ragaz.* Bad Ragaz: Privatdruck der Thermalbader und Grandhotels, 1970.

Schrödinger, Erwin. *What Is Life? and Mind And Matter.* London: Cambridge University Press, 1967.

Sewall, Richard B. Commencement Address, Walnut Hill School, Natick, Mass., June 6, 1975.

Shimkin, M. B. "Implementation of the Hospice Concept," in "Science and Cancer," a DHEW publication (NIH) 15-568, 1973.°

Shephard, David A. E. "Principles and Practice of Palliative Care," *CMA Journal* (March 5, 1977), pp. 522-26. °

————, "Terminal Care: Towards An Ideal," *CMA Journal* (July 17, 1976), pp. 97-8. °

Simonton, O. Carl. "Management of the Emotional Aspects of Malignancy." Lecture June 14, 1974, University of Florida, Gainesville, Florida.

Snow, Lois Wheeler. *A Death With Dignity: When the Chinese Came.* New York: Random House, 1974.

Solzhenitsyn, A. *The Cancer Ward.* New York: Dial Press, 1968.

Spenser, Edmund. *Selected Poetry,* ed. William Nelson. New York: Random House, 1964.

"Standards of Care for the Terminally Ill," *Ars Moriendi* Convention Report, Columbia, Md., Nov., 1974. °

Steinberg, Marion. "Death With Dignity," *The Journal of the Connecticut Business and Industry Association,* 54:11 (Nov., 1976). °

Steinfels, Peter and Robert M. Veatch, eds. *The Hastings Center Report: Death Inside Out.* New York: Harper, 1974.

Strauss, Anselm L. "Problems of Death and the Dying Patient," in *Aging in Modern Society,* edited by Alexander Simon and Leon J. Epstein. Washington: American Psychiatric Association, 1968.

Strauss, Maurice B., ed. *Familiar Medical Quotations.* Boston: Little, Brown, 1968.

Sudnow, David. *Passing On: The Social Organization of Dying in the County Hospital.* Englewood: Prentice-Hall, 1967.

Tennyson, Lord Alfred. *Idylls of the King.* New York: Airmont, 1969.

"Terminal Care: Connecticut Corp. Will Build a Hospital for the Dying," *Modern Health Care* (July, 1974), p. 101f. °

"The History of St. Barnabas' Home," (pamphlet). Worthing, England: St. Barnabas' Home. °

"The Hospice: An Alternative," *JAMA,* 236:18 (Nov. 1, 1976), p. 2047.°

Thomas, Lewis. *The Lives of A Cell.* New York: Viking, 1974.

Thompson, John D. and Grace Goldin. *The Hospital: A Social And Architectural History.* New Haven: Yale University Press, 1975.

Tolstoy, Leo. *The Death of Ivan Ilych and Other Stories.* New York: New American Library, 1960.

Toynbee, Arnold, Arthur Koestler, and others, eds. *Life After Death.* New York: McGraw-Hill, 1976.

Tozer, Eliot. "Hospices," *Practical Psychology For Physicians,* (Sept., 1976), pp. 61-67. °

Troup, Stanley B. and William A. Greene, eds. *The Patient, Death and the Family.* New York: Scribner, 1974.

Twycross, R. G., "Choice of Strong Analgesic in Terminal Cancer: Diamorphine or Morphine?" *Pain* (The Journal of the International Association for the Study of Pain) 3:2 (April, 1977), pp. 93-104. °

———, "Clinical Experience With Diamorphine in Advanced Malignant Disease," (reprint) *International Journal of Clinical Pharmacology,* 9:184. °

———, "Diseases of the Central Nervous System: Relief of Terminal Pain," (reprint) *British Medical Journal,* Oct. 25, 1975. °

———, "Principles and Practice of the Relief of Pain in Terminal Cancer," (reprint) *Update,* July, 1972. °

———, "Stumbling Blocks in the Study of Diamorphine," *Postgraduate Medical Journal* (May, 1973), pp. 309-13. °

———, "The Dying Patient," (pamphlet). London: CMF Publications, 1975. °

———, "The Terminal Care of Patients With Lung Cancer," *Postgraduate Medical Journal* (Oct., 1973), pp. 732-37. °

Verney, Richard E., ed. *The Student Life: The Philosophy of Sir William*

Osler. Edinburgh: Livingstone, 1952.

Wald, Florence S. "For Everything There is a Season and a Time to Every Purpose," *The New Physician* (April, 1969), pp. 278-85. °

Wentzel, K. B. "Dying Are The Living: St. Christopher's Hospice, London," *American Journal of Nursing,* 76:956-7 (Jan., 1976). °

Wessel. Morris A. "To Comfort Always," Yale Alumni Magazine, June, 1972, pp. 17-19. °

West. Thomas S. "Approach To Death," (reprint) *Nursing Mirror,* Oct. 10, 1974. °

———, "Hospice Care for a Dying Person and His Family." Paper presented at the First International Conference on Patient Counseling, Amsterdam, April, 1976. °

———, "The Final Voyage," *Frontier,* 17:4 (Winter, 1974). °

Woodward, Kenneth L. "There Is Life After Death," (an interview with Dr. Elisabeth Kübler-Ross), *McCall's* (August, 1976), pp. 97ff.

Worcester, A. *The Care of the Aged, the Dying and the Dead.* Springfield: Charles C. Thomas, 1961.

"Yale Plans Hospice Like St. Christopher's," *American Journal of Nursing* 71:2296 (December, 1971). °

Yates, Susan. "Experience With Dying Patients," *American Journal Of Nursing,* 73:6 (June, 1973). °

Xiques, Linda. "Dying At Home," (reprint) *Pacific Sun,* Jan, 28, 1977. °

Index